Information Circular 9477

Mining Roof Bolting Machine Safety: A Study of the Drill Boom Vertical Velocity

By Dean H. Ambrose, John R. Bartels, August J. Kwitowski, Raymond F. Helinski, Sean Gallagher, Ph.D., Linda J. McWilliams, and Thomas R. Battenhouse, Jr.

DEPARTMENT OF HEALTH AND HUMAN SERVICES
Centers for Disease Control and Prevention
National Institute for Occupational Safety and Health
Pittsburgh Research Laboratory
Pittsburgh, PA

May 2005

CONTENTS

ILLUSTRATIONS

Page

TABLES

TABLES–Continued

UNIT OF MEASURE ABBREVIATIONS USED IN THIS REPORT

fL	footlambert	in/sec	inch per second
ft	foot	lb	pound
hr	hour	msec	millisecond
in	inch	sec	second

MINING ROOF BOLTING MACHINE SAFETY: A STUDY OF THE DRILL BOOM VERTICAL VELOCITY

By Dean H. Ambrose,[1] John R. Bartels,[2] August J. Kwitowski,[3]
Raymond F. Helinski,[4] Sean Gallagher, Ph.D.,[5] Linda J. McWilliams,[6]
and Thomas R. Battenhouse, Jr.[7]

ABSTRACT

This report examines the boom arm vertical speed for roof bolting machines to study a moving boom arm appendage at different speeds during different work scenarios. The goal of this study is to determine the impact of the appendage speed on the likelihood of the operator's hand, arm, head, or leg making contact, such as touching the moving appendage. The overall research goal is to reduce workers' risks to injury from exposure to underground mining machinery.

Accident investigation reports from the Mine Safety and Health Administration do not usually contain enough information to aid in studying this problem, and lab experiments with human subjects are not feasible because of safety issues. As an alternative, researchers used a unique computer simulation model that uses a virtual human, vision tracking, and generates random virtual human motions and risky work behaviors. By using specialized software to simulate the computer model, researchers accurately identified potential hazards of tasks where it is not possible to perform experiments with human subjects.

Results of a frequency distribution analytic approach show that, regardless of other variables, contact incidents were always greater when the boom was moving up, always greater on the hand, and always greater for the boom arm part of the machine. The reason why the subject experiences more contacts when the boom arm is moving up rather than down is that more risky behaviors occur during drilling and bolting when the boom is ascending.

Results of a cross-tabulation analytic approach show that the 25th-percentile operators experienced more contacts than other operator sizes and had most of their contacts during a boom speed of 13 in/sec. The hand-on-boom behavior during drilling and bolting tasks experienced more contacts than other work behaviors, and both tasks had most of their contacts during speed 13 in/sec. The 60-in seam experienced more contacts than other seam heights and had most of the contacts during speed 16 in/sec.

For univariate logistic regression models, seam height is the most important predictor of the probability of a contact. However, a multivariate logistic regression model predicted contacts are more likely with the both-knee work posture in the 60-in seam, a 25th-percentile operator compared to a 55th-percentile operator, and speeds 16 and 22 in/sec compared to 7 in/sec.

Results of a survival analytic approach suggest that controlling the boom speed is the most important factor in determining the risk of an operator making contact. Based on the data collected, boom speeds greater than 13 in/sec result in a substantial increase in risk to the roof bolter operator making contact. Speeds less than or equal to 13 in/sec are associated with a more modest relative risk of making contact, which represents a decrease in potential hazard. Virtual operator's response time has little effect on the number of contacts experienced.

The mining industry can use the information in this study to reduce the likelihood that roof bolter operators will experience injury due to contact with a moving roof bolting machine's boom arm.

---

[1]Safety engineer, Pittsburgh Research Laboratory, National Institute for Occupational Safety and Health, Pittsburgh, PA.
[2]Mechanical engineer, Pittsburgh Research Laboratory, National Institute for Occupational Safety and Health, Pittsburgh, PA.
[3]Civil engineer, Pittsburgh Research Laboratory, National Institute for Occupational Safety and Health, Pittsburgh, PA.
[4]Electronics technician, Pittsburgh Research Laboratory, National Institute for Occupational Safety and Health, Pittsburgh, PA (retired).
[5]Research physiologist, Pittsburgh Research Laboratory, National Institute for Occupational Safety and Health, Pittsburgh, PA.
[6]Statistician, Pittsburgh Research Laboratory, National Institute for Occupational Safety and Health, Pittsburgh, PA.
[7]Geosciences system analyst, Science Applications International Corp., Augusta, GA.

INTRODUCTION

The Mine Safety and Health Administration's (MSHA) Health and Safety Accident Classification injury database showed an average of 660 roof bolter operator accidents per year over a 5-year period (1999–2003). This makes roof bolting the most hazardous machine-related job in underground mining, representing 39% of all machine-related accidents in underground coal mines. Protecting the safety of our Nation's mine workers is of paramount importance; however, there are currently no regulations or method of determining the safe speed of roof bolter boom arms. Several fatalities of operators of underground coal mining equipment have led to an investigation of safe vertical velocities of a roof bolter boom arm at the National Institute for Occupational Safety and Health's (NIOSH) Pittsburgh Research Laboratory (PRL). MSHA established a roof bolting machine committee with members from the West Virginia Board of Coal Mine Health and Safety, NIOSH, and roof bolter manufacturers. The committee's objective was to identify hazards and recommend solutions. The data collection effort involved analysis of MSHA accident data, visits to underground mines to interview experienced roof bolting machine operators, discussions with roof bolting machine manufacturers, interviews with workers who were injured while performing roof bolting tasks, and reviews of research on roof bolting safety. The information-gathering and fact-finding efforts of the committee identified 10 roof bolting-related problems that may have contributed to or caused accidents while the operator was within the drill head or boom pinch-point area (see figure 1). Seven of the 10 problems presented were associated with moving appendages [MSHA 1994]. Emphasis was placed on hazards related to the movement of the boom arm of a roof bolting machine. A set of solutions for each problem was recommended to increase the safety of roof bolting operations [MSHA 1994]. MSHA [1994] also recommended additional safety measures such as reduced drill speed rate, allowing the operator to react and either stop machine movement or move clear of a closing pinch point. One major observation regarding this study was that there are no data on safe speeds for booms operating close to workers in confined environments such as an underground coal mine.

This study reports the initial step to define a safe speed range for a roof bolter's boom arm. MSHA accident investigation reports do not usually contain scientific information to aid in studying interactions between a machine and its operator. In addition, lab experiments with human subjects are not feasible because of safety and ethical issues. With this in mind, NIOSH researchers successfully developed a computer model that uses UGS PLM Solutions' Jack simulation software. The model generates data by means of simulation while altering several variables associated with the machine and its operator. These include coal seam height, the operator's anthropometry, work posture, choice of risky behavior, and the machine's appendage velocity. The resulting simulation database has been studied by researchers to investigate appendage speeds and decrease the

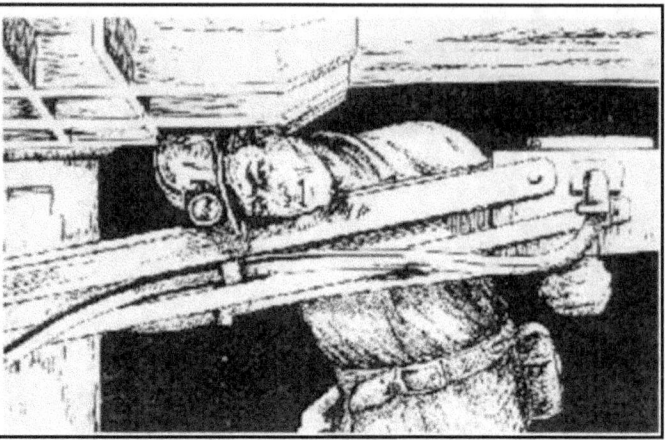

Figure 1. Artist concept of an operator caught within the boom arm and canopy.

number of contacts (possible injuries) to the miner by improving machine designs or operating procedures. Researchers believe that such simulations, treated with advanced statistical procedures such as logistic regression and survival analysis, provide very useful tools to evaluate the hazards of tasks where it is not possible to perform experiments with human subjects.

The model contains a virtual mine environment that includes roof bolter (figure 2) and operator models and experimentally mimics the virtual human and machine actions that can cause a contact. In this report, when operator limbs and a roof bolter appendage in the computer model interact and result in touching, the event is defined as a contact. Simulations of the model enable researchers to generate a database of contacts between a machine and its operator.

Three-dimensional computer simulations provide machine designers and safety analysts with a way to evaluate contact hazards concerning operator/machine interaction. Anthropos, Jack, Ramsis, and Safework are commercial software tools that digitally model humans for ergonomic analyses and work performance evaluations. NIOSH's simulator uses a roof bolting machine and biomechanical human models that execute on Jack (version 1.2) simulation software. Computer simulations enable the study of multiple mine environments (i.e., seams of different heights), motions of workers (represented by virtual humans), and different work scenarios (e.g., various drilling and bolting tasks, work postures, and risky work behaviors). These studies would be dangerous and time- and cost-prohibitive if they were conducted in the field.

One of the most difficult problems in using a computer simulator that generates human motions is trying to determine whether the model in the simulator accurately represents the actual mechanical system. The uncertainty and randomness inherent in a machine operator's tasks can be compared to someone drinking a beverage from a cup. Lifting the cup to one's mouth and placing it back onto the table exhibits some random variation in its motion path, and one could easily visualize the path of that motion. To model this random motion, the sequence of someone drinking a beverage from a cup would recur until the cup is empty. Each motion path would differ slightly even though the motions basically look alike. Likewise, in the case of a machine operator, the operator's work behaviors, motions of each behavior, and motion paths associated with each motion behavior will have some degree of randomness despite the basic task sameness. Through careful study, researchers successfully incorporated within the roof bolter model the randomness of the operator's motion and path variance within that motion. This factor of randomness gives NIOSH's simulator the capability to realistically represent the operator's motions and work behaviors while executing any machine task. Ambrose [2000, 2001, 2004] and Volberg and Ambrose [2002] discuss in detail the development of random motions used in the roof bolter model.

Before collecting final simulation data, researchers used test results by Bartels et al. [2001, 2003] on the roof bolter model to validate and ensure that parameter assumptions made for the computer-based simulation conform to actual field practice. Training videos, in-mine observations and videos, and working with a bolter manufacturer and experts helped to determine actual bolting practice. Studies by Bartels et al. [2001, 2003] verified the operator's response times, task motions, and field of view relative to the roof bolter's boom arm. Human subject tests with a full-scale working mockup of a roof bolter boom arm (figure 3) were used to collect motion data that helped determine parameters for building valid and credible models. The roof bolter model requires input data that closely matches an actual machine operating characteristics (e.g., dimensions and speeds) as well as data that accurately reflect physical characteristics of the operator, such as how close to the moving boom arm he or she is to reach machine controls and insert the drill steel or bolt into the drill head (figure 4). Researchers obtained these data by using a motion tracking/capturing system using experienced United Mine Workers of America (UMWA) miners as subjects. The subjects performed prescribed tasks on the mockup that mimic bolting practices that did not include risky behaviors as described in this report. Researchers found no differences between test subjects' actual bolting practice and recommended practice (according to roof bolting training materials). During human subject data collection, risky behaviors invalidated a test session, resulting in rerunning the test.

Experiments in other industries have provided some evidence for resolving safe machine appendage speeds for reducing potential hazards. Industries using robots exhibit concern for guidelines for robotics safety. Etherton [1987] reports that 10 in/sec is a speed whereby humans could recognize and react to a perceived hazard in the system. In addition, the Occupational Safety and Health Administration (OSHA) [1987] reports that robot speeds for teach-and-repeat programming sessions are required to be slow. The current standard of the American National Standards Institute recommends that this slow speed should not exceed 10 in/sec. However, Karwowski et al. [1992] report that test subjects with respect to the potential hazards

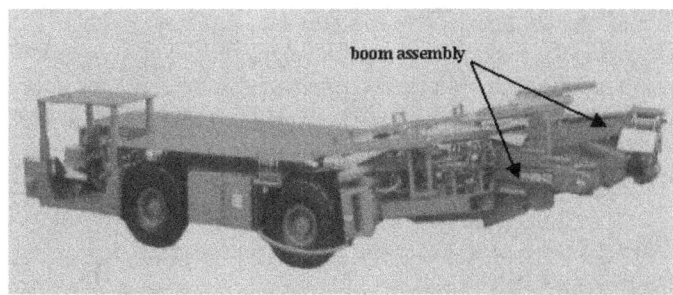

Figure 2. Actual dual boom arm roof bolting machine. (Photograph courtesy of J. H. Fletcher & Co., Huntington, WV.)

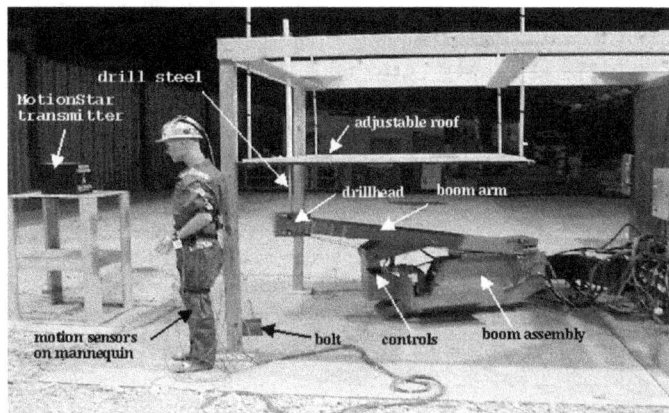

Figure 3. Full-scale wooden roof bolter boom arm setup for data collection. The mannequin illustrates motion sensor locations.

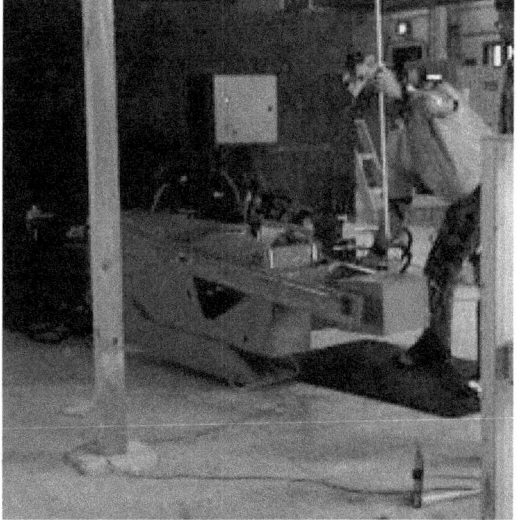

Figure 4. Operator close to the moving boom arm with hand on the controls.

from a moving robot arm similarly perceive the range of slow speeds of robot motion from 8 to 16 in/sec. Their study suggests that the safe slow speed of robot motions for teaching and programming purposes lies somewhere between 10 and 8 in/sec, and for safe reduced speed of robot motions redefines the current recommendation of 10 in/sec. Moreover, the U.S.

Department of Energy [1998] states that because the teacher can be within the robot's restrictive envelope, mistakes in programming can result in unintended movement, so a restricted speed of 6 in/sec is required on any part of the robot. This slower speed would minimize potential injuries to a teacher if inadvertent action or movement occurred.

This report documents NIOSH's success in achieving its expected outcome to examine the speed range of a roof bolter boom arm for different workplace scenarios and compare statistically which scenarios are most likely to cause contacts (possible injuries) to miners.

BACKGROUND

Roof bolting is one of the most basic functions and most dangerous jobs in underground coal mining. Roof bolts are the main method of roof support in mines, which is essential to ventilation and safety. After miner crews remove a section of the coal seam, roof bolting machine operators install bolts (steel rods) to secure areas of unsupported roof from caving in. A bolter crew's typical work sequence includes tramming and positioning the machine, general preparation and setup, drilling a hole, and installing a bolt. General preparation is a miscellaneous category that includes setting up temporary roof supports, scaling, handling ventilation material, performing a methane check, handling supplies, emptying the dust box, and examining the workplace. Drilling bolt holes involves inserting the drill steel in the chuck, adding extension steels if necessary, changing the bits, drilling the hole, and removing the steel. Bolt installation involves making up bolt assemblies, inserting resins in the hole if necessary, bending bolts, inserting bolts into the hole, aligning the bolts, raising bolts, and spinning to mix resin or torque the installed bolt. The sequence repeats until the assigned area of the roof is secure and then the machine trams to a new location.

Roof bolting may be regarded as a fairly structured and repetitive work situation. Although there is an established work cycle, it is commonly altered due to external influences, including variability in geology, interruption by coworkers and supervisors, machine malfunctions, variability of supplies, etc. The roof bolter operator is under constant production pressure to install as many bolts in one 8-hr shift as necessary to keep up with coal-cutting operations while remaining vigilant to all of the possible dangers. Consequently, roof bolting work in a newly exposed roof area involves even greater risk from the yet unsupported and unknown conditions.

The roof bolter operator does his or her job in a confined environment (see figure 5) in a limited working height, e.g., 45 in, and in close proximity and in low visibility to a moving drill head mounted on a boom arm 72 in long. This restricted work environment can force the operator in awkward postures for tasks that require quick reactions to avoid being contacted by moving machine parts. Restricted visibility due to a protection canopy and low lighting conditions further complicate the task. Moreover, roof bolters work in a newly exposed roof area; consequently, there is greater risk from the unsupported and unknown conditions.

The range of the operator location is about 20 to 38 inches from the boom arm because of the restricted work space or work posture when performing the bolting tasks. This range of distance brings the operator close to the boom arm while it is moving. Subsequently, this closeness allows the operator to easily reach the controls and perform tasks that require handling the drill steel and bolt that attaches to the drill head located at one end of the boom arm.

One major observation regarding the study by MSHA [1994] was that there are no data on safe speeds for booms operating close to workers in confined environments such as an underground coal mine. To address this problem, the main question that needs to be answered is: What range of boom speeds minimizes the roof bolter operator's chances of contact or possible injury without sacrificing job performance? This question becomes even more important in light of potential rules being discussed by MSHA on improving the design of roof bolters. The information needed to answer the question is—

• When does the operator see the moving boom arm and drill head during the bolting operation?
• How frequent are the contacts between the operator and moving machine appendages?
• What are the distances between the operator's hands, arms, legs, and head and the moving boom arm and drill head during each of the operator's job tasks?

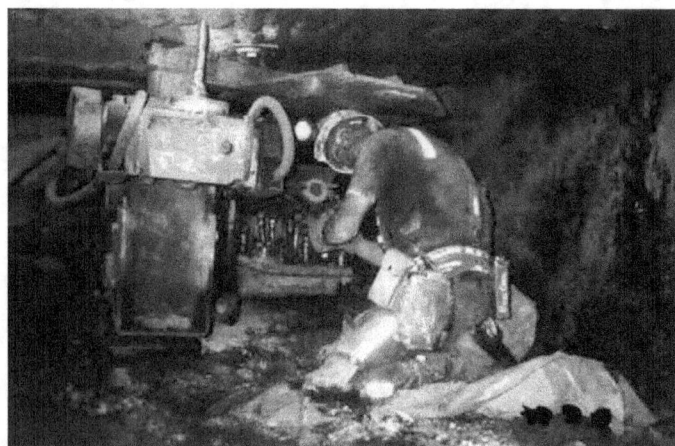

Figure 5. A roof bolter operator's work posture in an underground coal mine.

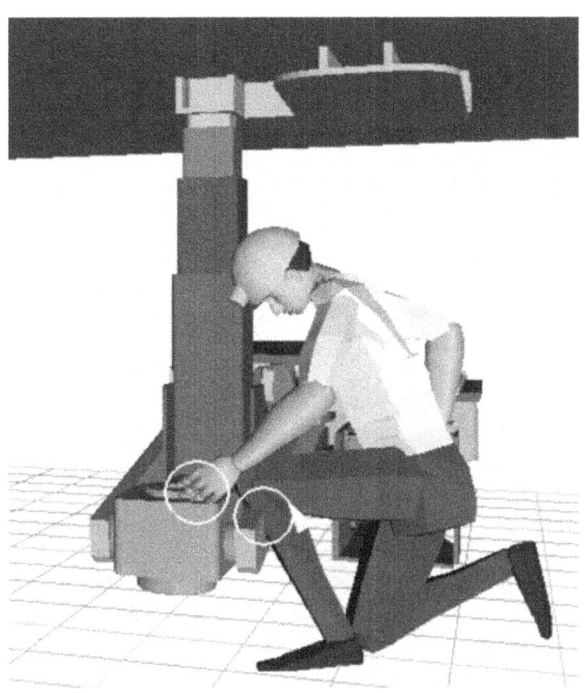

Figure 6. Virtual operator contacted in the left hand (or fingers) and left leg.

• How do changes in various work postures, such as kneeling on one knee, kneeling on two knees, or standing, impact the previous three questions?

To answer these questions effectively, a sufficient number of studies must be done to collect data on contacts and variables that influence them. A contact means the boom arm touches the operator's hand, arm, head, or leg (figure 6). A contact does not necessarily mean an injury. However, a severe injury or fatality can occur if the operator makes contact while in a drill head or boom arm pinch-point area. MSHA accident investigation reports do not usually contain enough information to aid in studying this particular problem, and lab experiments with human subjects are not feasible because of safety issues. Therefore, a computer simulation model approach was used as the primary means to generate and collect the data during boom arm movement [Ambrose 2000].

Previous studies by Klishis et al. [1993a,b] on worker job performance and machinery and work environment identified miners' risks and hazard exposures while bolting. More than two dozen bolting-related problems (including specific human behaviors) were recognized as potential situations that could lead to injury or expose workers to injury. Approaches to avoid these situations were suggested and applied at mining operations to evaluate specific problems in roof bolting tasks. Turin et al. [1995] conducted a human factors analysis of hazards related to the movement of the drill head boom of a roof bolting machine. Seven short-term recommendations to increase the safety of roof bolting operations were developed: use a dead-man interlock device to cut off power to the controls when the operator is out of position, place fixed barriers at pinch points and other dangerous areas, provide better control guarding, reduce the fast-feed speed, use automatic cutoff switches for pinch points and other dangerous areas, redesign the control bank to conform to accepted ergonomic principles, and use resin insertion tools and resin cartridge retainers.

RESEARCH

STUDY POPULATION

The study population used in the simulation software for any virtual human model can cover the 5th through 95th percentile for males and females. Using the wide-range capability of Jack software to scale the operator's anthropometry, researchers made three virtual operators that conformed to 25th-, 55th-, and 92nd-percentile males (table 1). The three virtual human models were chosen to match closely to human subject data that were collected for model verification/validation and to study the target population, which is 99% male. Since the goal of the lab tests was not to duplicate the entire simulation population but only to verify that the simulation model represents an accurate picture of the roof bolter model, a small sample of 12 human subjects from the local UMWA office was tested. Two female miners were study volunteers that represented 20th- to 30th-percentile male operators. Table 1 provides information on the height, weight, age, and sex for the 12 subjects used in the motion studies. The optimum viewing area tests used 12 subjects from NIOSH-PRL since no special mining skill was involved and no anthropometry data were needed.

MODEL VALIDATION

Two different methods to validate the model were chosen. The first method was the traditional face validity evaluation by roof bolter manufacturers and users. A questionnaire was developed and distributed to manufacturers, bolter operators, and mine inspectors. The responders were shown two animations that showed an operator performing roof bolting tasks: one was the virtual operator produced from the motion-capture data, the other was the virtual operator created from the model. The respondents were asked to compare aspects of the animations without knowing which motion source was shown in the animation by scoring on a scale from 4 being good to 1 being poor. The virtual operator produced from the motion-capture data scored an average of 2.55, the virtual operator created from the model scored an average of 2.34, and the average difference in questionnaire scoring was 0.64. Verification of the validity of the model was first implied when 14 of 15 responders agreed that the simulation animations did not differ significantly from the animations of human operators.

Table 1. Subject anthropometric data

Subject	Height, in	Weight, lb	Age, years	Sex	Operator percentile	Percentile interval
virtual25	66.4	159.4		male	24	20 30
virtual55	70.0	172.4		male	54	50 60
virtual92	71.8	187.0		male	91	90 95
human 1	71.0	187.2	47	male	84	80 90
human 2	68.7	135.8	54	male	51	50 60
human 3	69.4	177.7	41	male	61	60 70
human 4	69.2	179.5	44	male	58	50 60
human 5	70.4	185.9	49	male	79	70 80
human 6	71.9	194.0	49	male	92	90 95
human 7	66.5	169.8	53	female	24 (male)	20 30
human 8	66.4	168.5	47	female	24 (male)	20 30
human 9	69.7	183.9	50	male	63	60 70
human 10	71.8	198.2	47	male	91	90 95
human 11	69.3	183.0	44	male	59	50 60
human 12	68.3	174.9	48	male	49	40 50

Table 2. Data that met the acceptance criteria

Work posture	Condition	Percent met criteria
Both knees	60 in seam average operator	71.43
Both knees	60 in seam human subject operator	63.54
Right knee	60 in seam average operator	71.07
Right knee	60 in seam human subject operator	62.29
Standing	72 in seam average operator	69.64
Standing	72 in seam human subject operator	72.66
Starting position	Average operator	80.35
Starting position	Human subject operator	72.22
Overall average ..		70.40

The second method compared the motions generated by the simulation with motion data collected on human subjects. Although the predictions of the model could not be directly compared, the accuracy of the movements used to generate "contact data" could be. The aspects of operator movements determined to be critical were the range of motion of operators and variation in those movements.

Two sets of simulation data were generated from motion data of the knee and standing work postures. The first used virtual operators with anthropometric measurements identical to those of the 12 human subjects tested. Here, the data were compared on a subject-to-subject basis. The second set used operators generated from Jack software in seven different anthropometric sizes. Researchers compared data to an average of the human subjects within a 10th- percentile range, e.g., the Jack-generated 55th-percentile operator was compared to the average of the subjects in the 50th-60th percentile range.

The human subject movement data tended to vary greatly from individual to individual, making it impractical for a direct comparison of each individual's exact path of movement. Because the amount of movement and the variation of movement were the primary concerns, the comparisons were made between the statistical ranges by using standard deviation of movement. Researchers developed two sets of test data to verify the model. One set compared Jack-generated operators' motions in each of the anthropometric size ranges with human subject data averaged for that range ("average" operator). The other set

compared an individual test subject's motions with a simulation using that subject's anthropometry ("human subject" operator). The criterion for acceptance of the simulation data was less than 1.6-in difference from the human subject data, the static positional accuracy of the motion-tracking system with the resolution settings used.

Table 2 shows the percentage of range of motion data by using standard deviations that met the acceptance criteria. The simulations run using average operators (generated from Jack software 25th-, 45th-, 55th-, 65th-, 75th-, 85th-, and 92nd-percentile persons) showed a greater percentage of standard deviation values that met the acceptance criteria. This would be expected since averaged standard deviation values were used as the input data for the simulation. In general, the percentage of agreement was good in relation to modeling a scenario with the complexity of roof bolting.

To assess the performance of the model, Bartels et al. [2003] report in detail the lab experiments and results that compared movements of the virtual human in the model to those of their test subject counterparts. The report also discusses the evaluation of human motion and response time data to duplicate accurately the skills and experience involved in operating mining equipment.

EXPERIMENTAL DESIGN

The roof bolting operation was broken down into specific tasks. Klishis et al. [1993b] observed the tasks and the amount of time spent on each task. The task list provided a guide in developing the experimental design for lab human subject tests and motion scenarios for the computer simulations.

Early phases of roof bolter model development used input parameter values that were guesses to allow development to progress. Consequently, limited lab experiments were necessary to determine input parameters (e.g., accurate field of vision, human response in roof bolting postures, human motion envelopes of body appendages, and initial work starting postures) for the roof bolter model and to validate the model and simulations.

The computer model generates and collects contact data between the machine and its virtual operator while recording predictor variables, such as the seam height, the operator's starting positions, operator work postures, risky work behaviors, anthropometry, and the machine appendage velocity. Data collected by the roof bolter model consist of counting the number of contacts and recording the time when a contact happens.

Collected data were recorded to a file for each simulation scenario execution. The first line in the file contained information on the seam height, work posture, boom arm speed, operator anthropometry, and operator work behaviors. Furthermore, the following information was recorded every 0.03 sec to the file:

- Simulated time(s)
- The operator's initial distance (in) from the boom arm
- The boom arm distance (in) from a reference point on the floor level
- Distance calculations (in) between eight viewing area reference points and a reference point on the boom arm to help determine when the operator sees the boom arm
- A number marking sequential contacts between limbs and machine appendage was recorded for each simulated frame.

The computer model contains seven variables having different levels. The *seam height* (three levels) consisted of 45, 60, and 72 in to accommodate the operator's *work posture* (four levels): right knee, left knee, both knees, and standing. Human subject motion tests provided data that defined models of virtual humans whose percentile interval ranged from the 24th to the 92nd. The operator's final *anthropometry* (3 levels+) conformed to 25th-, 55th-, and 92nd-percentile males. Researchers also collected operator's *starting locations* from the human subject motion test data and calculated unique starting location values for each subject as a function of the seam height and work postures in that seam. The *operator's risky behavior during drilling* and *bolt installation* each had four levels. The five levels of the *boom arm speeds*—7, 10, 13, 16, and 22 in/sec—were selected from MSHA [1994]. Researchers had originally planned to collect data on four speeds. Based on initial results from the data analysis of a four-speed database, researchers could not speak to the risks associated with speeds between 10 and 16 in/sec. Therefore, researchers included a fifth speed, 13 in/sec, which split the difference between two initial speed levels.

A behavior motion is a series of human motions that mimics a specific action. Studies on worker job performance and machinery and work environment identify miners' risky work behavior and hazard exposures while bolting [Klishis et al. 1993a,b]. Researchers used this information to identify specific risky behaviors for the drilling operation and bolt installation (see table 3 and figures in appendix G). Also, researchers were interested in work behaviors occurring only when the machine appendage had movement; consequently, other risky behaviors associated with operating a roof bolter were not used. Ambrose's [2004] decision algorithm was integrated within the model that randomly selects which behavior to use for a simulation execution. Numerical parameters used in the algorithm came

from the percentage of operator actions that resulted in hazard exposure. These parameters were based on statistical observations of bolter operator actions associated with unsafe acts [Klishis et al. 1993a].

Table 3. Behavior list for drilling a hole and installing a bolt

Operation	Work behavior description
Drill	Hand off the drill steel and hand off the boom arm.
	Hand on the drill steel.
	Hand on the boom arm.
	Hand on the drill steel and then hand on the boom arm.
Bolt	Hand off the bolt or wrench and hand off the boom arm.
	Hand on the bolt or wrench.
	Hand on the boom arm.
	Hand on the bolt or wrench and then hand on the boom arm.

NOTE. Klishis et al. [1993a,b] were not specific with regard to hand location on the boom arm, drill steel, or wrench. In the simulations, researchers placed the hand on the boom arm approximately aft end of the drill head and placed the hand on drill steel, bolt, or wrench approximately midsection of the item.

As part of the experiment design, the operator's chance of avoiding a contact was also evaluated to ensure that an avoid incident (near-miss) would not be considered a contact. This required knowledge of when the operator sees the moving boom arm and the reaction time needed to avoid the boom arm. Investigators used information from Helander et al. [1987], Kobrick [1965], and Welford and Brebner [1980] to define a predetermined human response time— 250 msec (fast) and 400 msec (slow)—to get out of the way of a moving boom arm once it is seen. Table 4 quantifies data to determine "fast" and "slow" reaction times of operators as a function of seam height, work posture, and operators' anthropometric data.

Investigators originally used a viewing area for the virtual operator that was a cone with an oval directrix as defined by Humantech [2003] to experiment with the virtual human's vision-tracking capabilities. For acceptable viewing in reduced lighting conditions found in underground mines, MSHA's minimum lighting requirements mandate illumination levels of 0.06 fL. The viewing area was modified from lab test results on human subjects that determined the optimal viewing area and accurate field of vision for the virtual human in underground mines (figure 7).

Because investigators did not have access to the simulation software source code, the operator's reaction time in combination with the viewing area could not be made an integral part of the computer model. Consequently, when executing simulations, recorded data included time of contacts and when the boom arm was in and out of the operator's view. Subsequently, during data postprocessing of the contact database, a collision check algorithm compared time-pairings of when the boom arm was in and out of view to determine suspected avoid incidents (near-misses). The results provided investigators with enough information that identified contacts that could be avoided by the operator.

The 25th-, 55th-, and 92nd-percentile operator models were placed in a virtual mine environment that contained a model of

Table 4. Reaction times of operators used in the roof bolter model, milliseconds

| Operator percentile | 45 IN SEAM HEIGHT | | | | | |
| | Right knee work posture | | Left knee work posture | | Both knees work posture | |
	Fast reaction time	Slow reaction time	Fast reaction time	Slow reaction time	Fast reaction time	Slow reaction time
25th	436	736	356	656	376	676
55th	401	701	366	666	397	697
92nd	330	630	384	684	349	649

| Operator percentile | 60 IN SEAM HEIGHT | | | | | |
| | Right knee work posture | | Left knee work posture | | Both knees work posture | |
	Fast reaction time	Slow reaction time	Fast reaction time	Slow reaction time	Fast reaction time	Slow reaction time
25th	370	670	376	676	356	656
55th	333	633	392	692	353	653
92nd	403	703	424	724	375	675

| Operator percentile | 72 IN SEAM HEIGHT | |
| | Standing work posture | |
	Fast reaction time	Slow reaction time
25th	374	674
55th	376	676
92nd	388	688

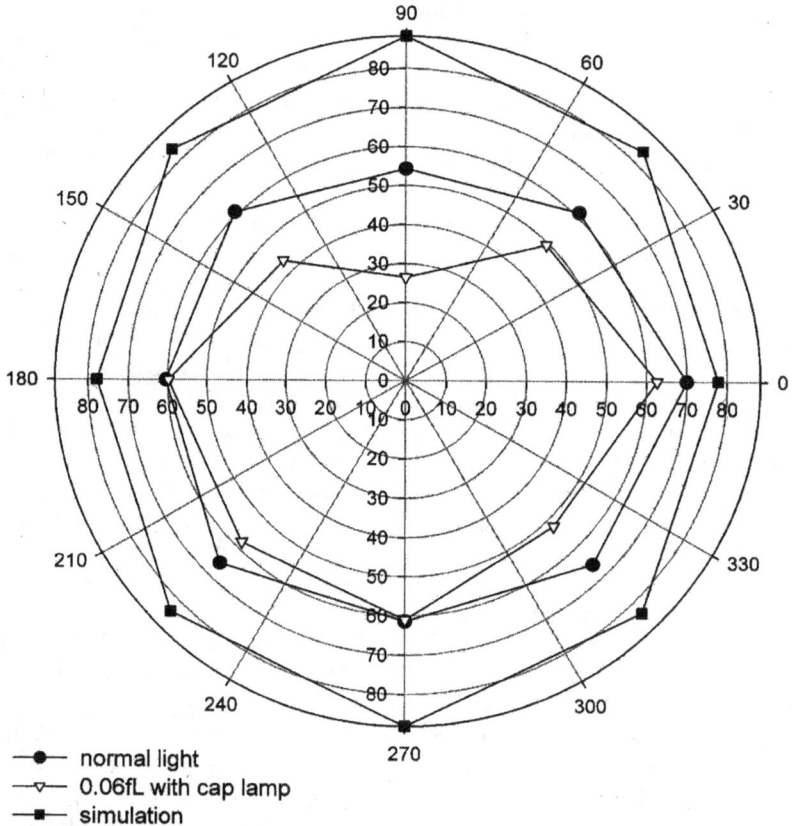

—●— normal light
—▽— 0.06fL with cap lamp
—■— simulation

Figure 7. Angular data of the original and modified viewing areas for the virtual operator.

a Fletcher[8] roof bolter boom arm assembly. When using the virtual mine environment, simulations were executed on each percentile operator while performing 1 of 35 possible scenarios (table 5). For example, simulation scenario 17 (in table 5) is one observation for any percentile operator who performs bolting tasks in a seam height of 60 in, on the left knee, and with a boom arm operating at a speed of 7 in/sec. The scenarios consisted of various combinations of the seam height, work posture, and boom arm speed. Researchers did not simulate the standing work posture in the two lower seam heights. Also, the knee work postures were not simulated in the highest seam height. When simulating any scenario, each simulation execution represented one observation, and information for that observation was recorded to one data file.

[8]J. H. Fletcher & Co. was a project collaborator. Fletcher provided information on a roof bolting machine. The company is the largest U.S. manufacturer of roof bolting equipment.

Table 5. Thirty-five possible simulation scenarios for each operator percentile

Scenario	Seam height, in			Work posture				Boom speed, in/sec				
	45	60	72	Right knee	Left knee	Both knees	Standing	7	10	13	16	22
1	✔			✔				✔				
2	✔				✔			✔				
3	✔					✔		✔				
4	✔			✔					✔			
5	✔				✔				✔			
6	✔					✔			✔			
7	✔			✔						✔		
8	✔				✔					✔		
9	✔					✔				✔		
10	✔			✔							✔	
11	✔				✔						✔	
12	✔					✔					✔	
13	✔			✔								✔
14	✔				✔							✔
15	✔					✔						✔
16		✔		✔				✔				
17		✔			✔			✔				
18		✔				✔		✔				
19		✔		✔					✔			
20		✔			✔				✔			
21		✔				✔			✔			
22		✔		✔						✔		
23		✔			✔					✔		
24		✔				✔				✔		
25		✔		✔							✔	
26		✔			✔						✔	
27		✔				✔					✔	
28		✔		✔								✔
29		✔			✔							✔
30		✔				✔						✔
31			✔				✔	✔				
32			✔				✔		✔			
33			✔				✔			✔		
34			✔				✔				✔	
35			✔				✔					✔

Table 6 shows how the simulation executions were organized into test series called data sets. The test series helped researchers with distributing the work in gathering data from simulation executions. Data sets were developed by using all of the simulation scenarios reflected in table 5. A data set contains a fixed seam height, boom arm speed, operator work posture, and anthropometry. Furthermore, data sets were also used to help show results in frequency data analysis.

Table 7 summarizes the factors (per seam height) that were used to generate observations (data files) that made up the research database. Note that the database represents the equivalence of actual field observations of roof bolting work in underground coal mines for a period of 12.15 eight-hour shifts. The 8-hr shift data were calculated using information from an unpublished time study of a roof bolter cycle time that installed 4-ft bolts with a dual-boom bolter equipped with an automatic temporary roof support system. The roof bolter equipment in the time study was the same machine model and bolt length used in the simulation.

MEASUREMENTS

Virtual human models that matched closely to human subject data collected for model verification/validation were given specific instructions as to how to perform the bolting tasks for each of the simulation scenarios. In each condition, the virtual operator was required to work in the starting posture throughout the tasks. Three kneeling postures were used in the two lower seam heights. The standing posture was used in the unrestricted (high) seam. The standing postures for the two taller operators were flexing more toward the right side and forward to accommodate the workspace and proper right-hand alignment with the machine controls. This posturing was also observed during lab tests that collected human subject motion data for validating the model. The random starting position between the operator and boom arm were based on seam height and the operator's work posture according to results from human subject lab tests. Each virtual operator faced perpendicular to the long side of the boom arm, and the machine controls were always to

Table 6. Data sets composed of conditions, operator percentile, and assigned numbering scheme

Conditions[1]	Operator percentile	Execution's assigned number range		Conditions[1]	Operator percentile	Execution's assigned number range		Conditions[1]	Operator percentile	Execution's assigned number range	
4507R	25th	0000	0049	6007R	25th	1800	1849	7207S	25th	3600	3649
	55th	0050	0099		55th	1850	1899		55th	3650	3699
	92nd	0100	0149		92nd	1900	1949		92nd	3700	3749
4507L	25th	0150	0199	6007L	25th	1950	1999	7210S	25th	3750	3799
	55th	0200	0249		55th	2000	2049		55th	3800	3849
	92nd	0250	0299		92nd	2050	2099		92nd	3850	3899
4507B	25th	0300	0349	6007B	25th	2100	2149	7216S	25th	3900	3949
	55th	0350	0399		55th	2150	2199		55th	3950	3999
	92nd	0400	0449		92nd	2200	2249		92nd	4000	4049
4510R	25th	0450	0499	6010R	25th	2250	2299	7222S	25th	4050	4099
	55th	0500	0549		55th	2300	2349		55th	4100	4149
	92nd	0550	0599		92nd	2350	2399		92nd	4150	4199
4510L	25th	0600	0649	6010L	25th	2400	2449	4513R	25th	4200	4249
	55th	0650	0699		55th	2450	2499		55th	4250	4299
	92nd	0700	0749		92nd	2500	2549		92nd	4300	4349
4510B	25th	0750	0799	6010B	25th	2550	2599	4513L	25th	4350	4399
	55th	0800	0849		55th	2600	2649		55th	4400	4449
	92nd	0850	0899		92nd	2650	2699		92nd	4450	4499
4516R	25th	0900	0949	6016R	25th	2700	2749	4513B	25th	4500	4549
	55th	0950	0999		55th	2750	2799		55th	4550	4599
	92nd	1000	1049		92nd	2800	2849		92nd	4600	4649
4516L	25th	1050	1099	6016L	25th	2850	2899	6013R	25th	4650	4699
	55th	1100	1149		55th	2900	2949		55th	4700	4749
	92nd	1150	1199		92nd	2950	2999		92nd	4750	4799
4516B	25th	1200	1249	6016B	25th	3000	3049	6013L	25th	4800	4849
	55th	1250	1299		55th	3050	3099		55th	4850	4899
	92nd	1300	1349		92nd	3100	3149		92nd	4900	4949
4522R	25th	1350	1399	6022R	25th	3150	3199	6013B	25th	4950	4999
	55th	1400	1449		55th	3200	3249		55th	5000	5049
	92nd	1450	1499		92nd	3250	3299		92nd	5050	5099
4522L	25th	1500	1549	6022L	25th	3300	3349	7213S	25th	5100	5149
	55th	1550	1599		55th	3350	3399		55th	5150	5199
	92nd	1600	1649		92nd	3400	3449		92nd	5200	5249
4522B	25th	1650	1699	6022B	25th	3450	3499				
	55th	1700	1749		55th	3500	3549				
	92nd	1750	1799		92nd	3550	3599				

[1]The first two digits represent seam height (in). The second two digits represent boom arm speed (in/sec). The letter represents work posture as follows: R = right knee; L = left knee; B = both knees; S = standing.

Table 7. Factors that determined the number of observations (simulation executions) per seam height

Observation totals	Seam height, in	Factors			
		Operators	Boom speeds	Work postures	Simulation executions
2,250	45	3	5	3	50
2,250	60	3	5	3	50
750	72	3	5	1	50
Overall 5,250					

Table 8. Sample data output file

CONF=1	SEAM=2	POST=3	SPED=1	SUBJ=1	BEHD=1	BEHB=1												
time	OPL	V1	V2	V3	V4	V5	V6	V7	V8	BAM	LPB	LPD	LAB	LAD	LLB	LLD	RLB	RLD	HDB
0.03	54.	4.	38.	5.	63.	28.	58.	32.	20.	19.	0.	0.	0.	0.	0.	0.	0.	0.	0.
0.06	54.	4.	38.	5.	63.	28.	58.	32.	20.	19.	0.	0.	0.	0.	0.	0.	0.	0.	0.
0.10	54.	4.	38.	5.	63.	28.	58.	32.	20.	19.	0.	0.	0.	0.	0.	0.	0.	0.	0.
0.13	54.	4.	38.	5.	63.	28.	58.	32.	20.	19.	0.	0.	0.	0.	0.	0.	0.	0.	0.
0.16	54.	4.	38.	5.	63.	28.	58.	32.	20.	19.	0.	0.	0.	0.	0.	0.	0.	0.	0.
0.20	54.	4.	38.	5.	63.	28.	58.	32.	20.	19.	0.	0.	0.	0.	0.	0.	0.	0.	0.
0.23	54.	4.	38.	5.	63.	28.	58.	32.	20.	19.	0.	0.	0.	0.	0.	0.	0.	0.	0.

First line and columns of data file (coded)	Subsequent lines and columns in data file

CONF machine control configuration
  1=piano key controls
SEAM seam height
  1=45 in; 2=60 in; 3=72 in
POST work posture
  1=right knee; 2=left knee; 3=both knees; 4=standing
SPED boom arm speed
  1=7 in/sec; 2=10 in/sec
  3=16 in/sec; 4=22 in/sec
  5=13 in/sec
SUBJ operator's anthropometry
  1=25th; 2=55th; 3=92nd
BEHD operator's behavior during the drilling task
  1=none; 2=hand on drill
  3=hand on boom; 4=hand on both
BEHB operator's behavior during the bolting task
  1=none; 2=hand on bolt
  3=hand on boom; 4=hand on both
	time simulated time, sec
	OPL operator's distance from the boom arm, in
	V1 through V8 reference points on the vision cone whose values are used to determine if the boom arm is seen by the operator
	BAM to determine boom arm movement, a distance is measured between a floor reference point and boom arm reference, in
	LPB through HDB a numerical marking that indicates if a contact occurred between an operator limb and machine appendage. "1" means contact; "0" means no contact.
	LPB / LPD = left palm with boom / with drill head
	LAB / LAD = left forearm with boom / with drill head
	LLB / LLD = left leg with boom / with drill head
	RLB / RLD = right leg with boom / with drill head
	HDB = head with boom arm

the operator's right. The virtual operator grabbed the tools (drill steel, bolt, or wrench) with the right hand, passed the tool off to the left hand, and grabbed them with both hands to finish setting the tool in the drill head and/or hole in the mine ceiling (mine roof).

Once the preparation for the drilling or bolt installation task was completed, the right hand was positioned on the appropriate lever that controlled the boom arm's vertical movement. Boom arm speed was the same ascending and descending. During the boom arm movement, the left hand's motion would be one of four possible risky work behaviors as defined in table 3. At no time during boom arm movement was the virtual operator positioned in a pinch-point area of the drill head or boom arm.

When the virtual operator and machine interacted and resulted in touching, the event was defined as a contact. Researchers were interested in contacts occurring only when the machine appendage was moving. Furthermore, the model included random operators' motions before and after the boom arm appendage moved [Ambrose 2004]. These motions helped to improve motion accuracy through random positioning of the arm and hand just before or after appendage movement. Also,

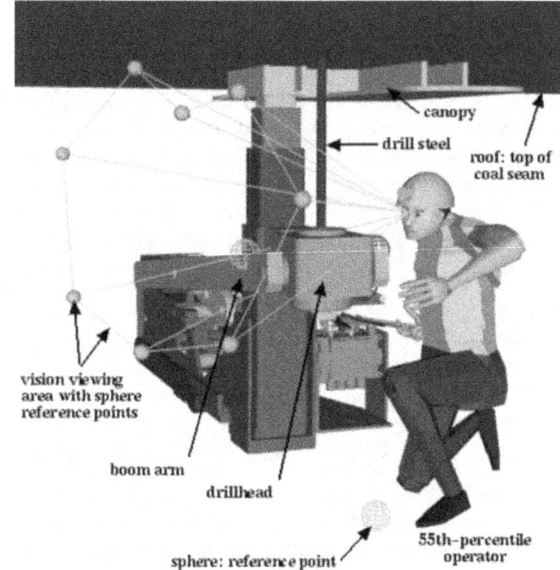

Figure 8. A view of the roof bolter model from a computer monitor.

these motions made the overall model (figure 8), when simulated, look visually realistic.

Data were collected according to the organized data sets (table 5). Three separate computers were used in the data-gathering phase of the study. Using different computers did not influence simulation outcomes because a copy of the simulation model executed perfectly on all computers. No changes or modifications to the model were necessary for any of the computers used in data collection. The data collection phase took 5 months to complete.

Researchers had each of the 5,250 simulation executions stored in separate data files. One data file contained lines of information identified by a timeframe. The number of timeframes varied because the length of a simulation execution changed due to one or more of the following: boom speed, seam height, or risky work behavior. A timeframe constitutes one line of data in the output file, except for the first line in the file, which describes each simulation scenario. Table 8 shows several lines of a data file. The table also includes definitions for line and column descriptors.

DATA ANALYSIS

Results of this analysis of roof bolter simulations provide information that could be quite helpful in making recommendations to reduce the likelihood that roof bolter operators get injured from contact with a moving boom arm. Researchers believe that the use of such simulations, treated with frequency and cross-tabulation and advanced statistical procedures such as logistic regression and survival analysis, provide extremely useful tools to evaluate potential hazards of tasks where it is not possible to perform experiments with human subjects.

NIOSH contracted with Science Applications International Corp. (SAIC), Augusta, GA, to assist in the data-postprocessing phase of the research. SAIC postprocessed data from 5,250 simulation executions with the aid of a customized software program whose algorithm followed the flow diagram in figure 9. SAIC generated the final database by developing a customized program based on NIOSH's algorithm that detailed sequences for examining the simulation results. NIOSH analysts used SAIC's final database for this portion of the study.

The resulting database contains information representing variables that could influence predictions of contact incidents between the operator's body parts and the moving boom arm and drill head. The determinations of contact incidents for each simulation execution resulted in four possible occurrences:

• A contact between the machine and the operator for a person with both slow and fast reactions.
• A contact between the machine and the operator for a person with only slow reactions.
• An avoid incident (near-miss) where a contact occurred in the simulation, but postanalysis determined that the operator saw the bolter boom arm and had fast enough reactions to get out of the way of (avoid) the contact.
• A complete simulation execution where no contacts or avoid incidents occurred (none).

A simulation execution would continue to completion even though it was possible for a single simulation to have multiple contacts and avoids. The presence of multiple incidents in a single simulation execution meant that data analysis could be done on either a data set containing avoids and all contacts (all of the contacts) or one incident per simulation execution (one run/one contact). Consequently, researchers made two separate sets of data from the initial postprocessed database.

Table 9 compares the two sets of data. This comparison showed that the source of contact incidents and the relationship of the variables associated with the incidents did not differ significantly for the two. The one run/one contact data set was also considered by researchers to more accurately represent the real-world situation, as an operator would most likely stop or at least pause after being struck with a moving machine appendage. The one run/one contact data set also lent itself to other types of data analysis techniques such as logistic regression and survival analysis.

Analysis also shows that the reaction time of the operator did *not* significantly affect the outcome of the simulation (table 10). The number of contact incidents for an operator with slow reactions differed from those for an operator with fast reactions by less than 1% in both data sets. The results were as expected insofar as there was a difference. There was a reasonable difference in reaction times between fast and slow operators obtained from reaction time tests on our human subjects. However, the speculation as to why a small difference in contacts might be reflected in the speed range of the boom being studied is that if the operator with fast reactions could not get out of the path of the boom, the slower operator certainly would not either. Also, depending on the stimulus, small differences were found in some reaction time test cases in the literature search. Moreover, literature reviews were not helpful with whole-body reaction of the upper torso and limbs in confined spaces, which was a concern in our research.

The following sections contain frequency and cross-tabulation, logistic regression, and survival analyses. All analyses were conducted using only the occurrences for the operator with slow reactions that included one contact per simulation executions (one run/one contact). Frequency analysis is the simplest method to observe how different categories of values are distributed in the sample database. Customarily, if a data set includes any categorical data (e.g., seam height, appendage speed, work posture, etc.), then one of the first steps in the data analysis is to compute a frequency table for those variables. Cross-tabulation is a combination of two (or more) frequency tables arranged such that each cell in the resulting table represents a unique combination of specific values of cross-tabulated variables. Thus, cross-tabulation allows researchers to examine frequencies of observations that belong to

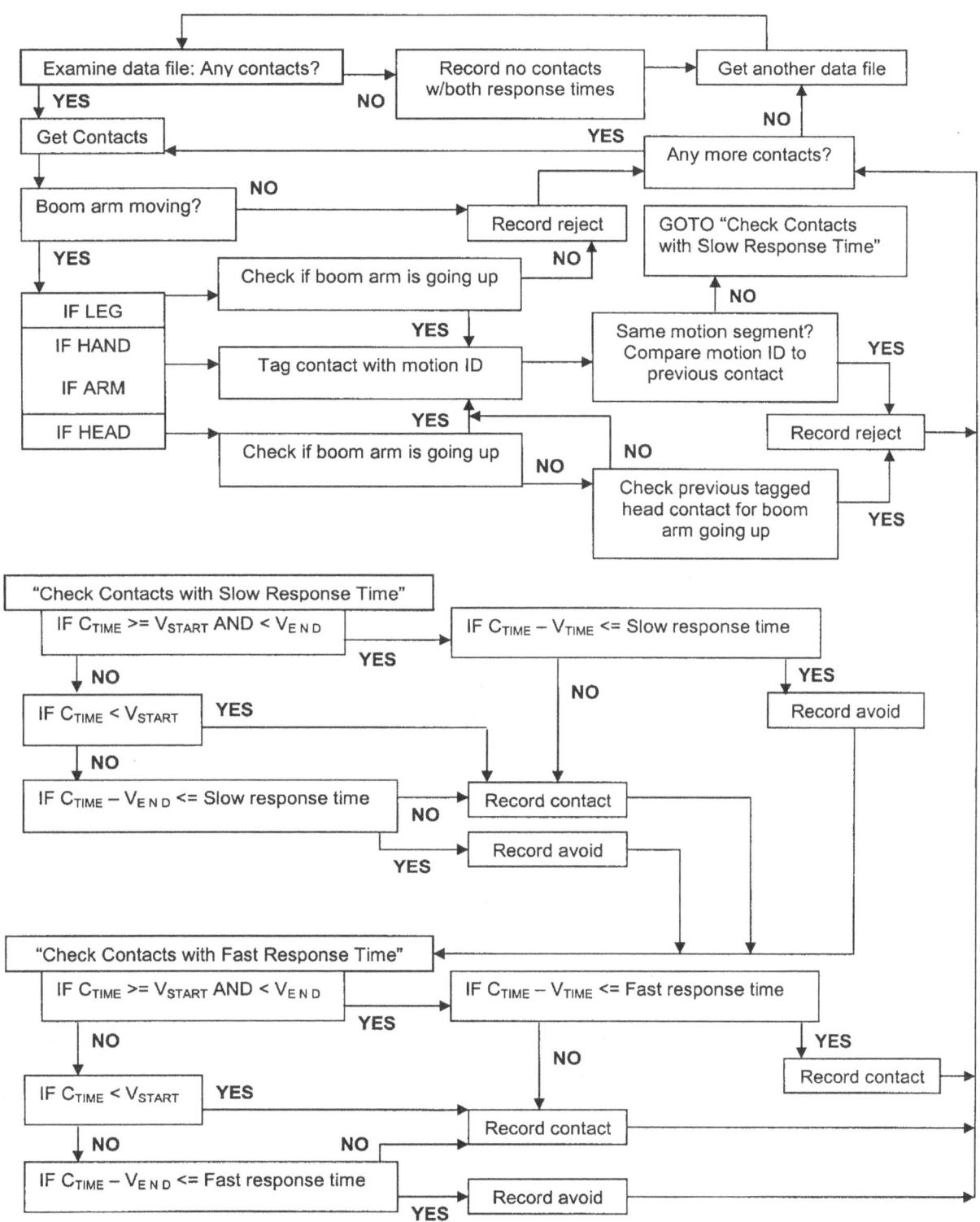

Figure 9. Flowchart of NIOSH's algorithm for processing the simulation data files.

Table 9. Comparison of one contact per execution versus all contacts

Variable	Reaction time	One run/one contact		All contacts	
		Avoid incidents	Contacts	Avoid incidents	Contacts
Seam height, in	Slow	45>60>72	60>45>72	60>45>72	60>72>45
	Fast	45>60>72	60>45>72	60>45>72	60>72>45
Operator percentile	Slow	92>55>25	25>55>92	25>55>92	25>55>92
	Fast	55>25>92	25>55>92	25>55>92	25>55>92
Work posture[1]	Slow	L>B>R>S	B>R>L>S	L>B>R>S	B>R>S>L
	Fast	L>B>R>S	B>R>L>S	L>B>R>S	B>R>L>S
Boom arm speed, in/sec	Slow	10>13>7>22>16	16>22>13>10>7	10>13>7>16>22	16>22>7>13>10
	Fast	10>13>7>22>16	16>22>7>10	10>13>7>16>22	16>22>7>13>10
Drilling behavior[2]	Slow	B>D&B>N>D	B>D&B>N>D	B>D&B>N>D	B>N>D&B>D
	Fast	B>D&B>N>D	B>N>D&B>D	B>D&B>N>D	B>N>D&B>D
Bolting behavior[3]	Slow	N>B>BT>BT&B	B>N>BT&B>BT	B>N>BT&B>BT	B>BT&B>N>BT
	Fast	B>N>BT>BT&B	B>N>BT&B>BT	B>N>BT&B>BT	B>BT&B>N>BT
Boom direction[4]	Slow	D>U	U>D	D>U	U>D
	Fast	D>U	U>D	D>U	U>D
Body part[5]	Slow	H>L>A>HD	H>L>HD>A	H>L>A>HD	H>A>L>HD
	Fast	H>L>A>HD	H>L>HD>A	H>L>A>HD	H>A>L>HD
Side[6]	Slow	L>R>HD	L>HD>R	L>R>HD	L>HD>R
	Fast	L>R>HD	L>HD>R	L>R>HD	L>HD>R
Machine part[7]	Slow	B>D	B>D	B>D	B>D
	Fast	B>D	B>D	B>D	B>D

[1]L = left knee; R = right knee; B = both knees; S = standing.
[2]B = hand on boom; D = hand on drill steel; D&B = hand on drill steel then on boom; N = none.
[3]B = hand on boom; BT = hand on bolt; BT&B = hand on bolt then on boom; N = none.
[4]D = down; U = up.
[5]H = hand; L = leg; A = arm; HD = head.
[6]L = left; R = right; HD = head.
[7]B = boom; D = drill head.

Table 10. Results of slow versus fast reaction for simulation executions

	All contacts			One contact per simulation		
	Frequency	Percent	Cumulative percent	Frequency	Percent	Cumulative percent
			SLOW OPERATOR			
Avoid	2,777	27.02	27.02	755	14.38	14.38
Contact	5,798	56.42	83.45	2,750	52.38	66.76
None	1,701	16.55	100.00	1,745	33.24	100.00
Total	10,276	100.00		5,250	100.00	
			FAST OPERATOR			
Avoid	2,768	26.94	26.94	799	15.22	15.22
Contact	5,807	56.51	83.45	2,706	51.54	66.76
None	1,701	16.55	100.00	1,745	33.24	100.00
Total	10,276	100.00		5,250	100.00	

specific categories for more than one variable. By examining these frequencies, researchers can identify relationships between cross-tabulated variables and provide information on trends to use other statistical approaches for the database.

Logistic regression is a technique used for relating one or more independent variables to an outcome variable, which follows a binomial rather than a normal distribution. This model is useful for identifying risk factors related to the presence or absence of a condition. Researchers used the logit (logistic) transformation of p (the probability of an event or nonevent) as the dependent variable. Complex numerical algorithms are generally required to fit the parameters of the model.

Survival analysis is a statistical technique that allows researchers to determine factors that influence both whether an event occurs (for example, contact between the boom and operator) and the time until that event occurs. In the present situation, this event might represent contact between the boom of the roof bolter and the worker operating the machine at some point in the period of a simulation execution. Since several variables (such as boom speed, work posture, worker behaviors, etc.) were varied in the simulations, survival analysis can be used to evaluate which of these factors were most important in terms of predicting an event (contact), as well as whether certain work behaviors, postures, or other factors might actually *protect* a worker from experiencing a contact.

Presenting various approaches to data analysis was part of the research objective, and each analysis technique used the same database. However, we do not recommend comparing results from each approach because of the differences in underlying mathematics, the computational details, and expected outcomes.

FREQUENCY AND CROSS-TABULATION ANALYSIS

Method

Variables Investigated

The model used three types of predictor variables: (1) fixed variables were used as input for simulation setup, (2) conditional variables were randomly selected within the computer model and then fixed before executing the simulation, and (3) random variables were "values" that changed during the simulation execution. The fixed variables were:

- *Roof bolter boom arm speed.*—The boom speeds used were 7, 10, 13, 16, and 22 in/sec. When the boom arm moved up or down for drilling or bolting, one selected speed was maintained for all events throughout the simulation execution.
- *Seam height.*—The area in which the operator had to perform the roof bolting procedure is defined as the distance from the floor to the top of the coal seam or roof, which may go beyond the top of the coal seam. The specific heights used were 45, 60, and 72 in.
- *Operator's posture while performing the roof bolting tasks.*—The work postures used were kneeling on the right knee, kneeling on the left knee, kneeling on both knees, and standing. The one selected work posture was maintained throughout the simulation execution.
- *Operator's anthropometry.*—The operators' percentiles were grouped within the general population as determined by height. The percentile size operators used were 25th, 55th, and 92nd.

The conditional variables were:

- *Operator's behavior during the drilling phase of the simulation.*—Drilling behavior was randomly selected before beginning the simulation. The operator could place his hand on the drill steel, place his hand on the boom arm, place his hand on the drill steel then the boom arm, or the hand would not be placed on any of the machine parts.
- *Operator's behavior during the bolting phase of the simulation.*— Bolting behavior was randomly selected before beginning the simulation. The operator could place his hand on the bolt, place his hand on the boom arm, place his hand on the bolt then the boom arm, or the hand would not be placed on any of the machine parts.
- *Operator's location.*—The operator would be randomly positioned with respect to the bolter at the beginning of the simulation. The operator location is defined as the distance from a reference point on the boom arm to a reference point in the small of the operator's back. At no time during boom arm movement was the operator positioned in pinch-point areas of the drill head or boom arm.

The random variables were:

- *Boom arm direction (up or down).*—This is the direction in which the boom arm was moving when an incident, either a contact or an avoid incident, occurred. The direction could only be one of two directions, up or down, and if the boom arm was not in motion the incident would not be used.
- *Body part (hand, arm, leg, and head).*—This is the part of the operator involved in an incident. The parts of the body that could potentially be struck by the moving boom arm were the hand, arm, leg, or head.
- *Machine part (boom arm and drill head).*—This is the part of the bolting machine assembly that could strike the operator. The only moving parts used for this simulation were the boom arm and drill head.

Data

Frequency and cross-tabulation analyses included 5,250 simulation executions. Of the simulations examined, 2,750 exhibited contact between the boom and the operator.

Results

Frequency Analysis

A table of incidents was compiled for fixed, conditional, and random variables used in the simulation in order to determine their effect on the operator (contacts between the operator and the machine). The results of the tabulation of incidents by variable showed which variables played the largest role in the occurrences of potential contacts to operators. The variables that were associated with the greatest number of contacts and avoid incidents are presented. The following appendices in this report contain charts and tables for frequency analysis: appendix A, "Frequency of Incidents"; appendix B, "Frequency by Operator Location"; and appendix C, "Frequency Data Sets."

Fixed Variables

As shown in table A–1, the 60-in seam height had the most contacts, 59% of the total number of contacts and 25% of the avoid incidents. Table A–2 shows that the anthropometry did not show a large difference for any one size individual, but the 25th-percentile operator had 40% of the total contact incidents. Table A–3 shows that the work posture on both knees had the greatest number of contact incidents compared to other postures (32% of the total contacts). Table A–4 shows that all boom arm speeds resulted in contact incidents; the faster speeds (16 and 22 in/sec) accounted for 43% of the total contacts.

Conditional Variables

Data in tables A–5 and A–6 show that the hand-on-boom behavior for drilling or bolting had more contacts than any other drilling or bolting behavior. Table B–1 showed three locations with increased contact incidents: 21.7, 29.9, and 30.3 in. Further sorting of operator location indicated that the increase at 21.7 in was associated with increased head incidents with the operator on both knees in a 60-in seam height (see tables B–2 to B–4). The increase in incidents at 29.9 and 30.3 in were associated with the operator in a standing position and an increase in contacts with the hand (see tables B–2 and B–3).

Random Variables

Table A–7 shows the boom arm upward direction had significantly more contacts (76% of the total) and fewer avoid incidents (37% of the total) than the down direction. Table A–8 shows the hand was involved in 67% of all contact incidents. Table A–9 shows the boom arm was the closest moving machine part to the operator and accounted for 80% of all contact incidents.

Data Sets

Frequency analysis was done on the data sets described in table 6. The data set for each simulation execution was a predetermined set of the variables assigned for a set of 50 simulation executions. An example of this would be 45R07, which defines the set of conditions for a 45-in seam height, with the operator on the right knee and the boom arm speed set at 7 in/sec. Examining the data sets in tables C–1 and C–2 confirms trends seen when the results for the individual variables were analyzed. Examples of this analysis show: (1) data sets 6022B and 6016B (60-in seam height with the operator on both knees) had the most contacts, (2) data sets 4510L and 4510B (45-in seam height with the operator on both knees) had the most avoid incidents, and (3) the hand for data set 7207S and the head for data set 6022B had the most contacts.

Cross-tabulation Analysis

A cross-tabulation of incidents was compiled for selected variables used in the simulation in order to determine their effect on contacts between the operator and machine. The results of the tabulation of contact incidents by variable showed which variables played the largest role in the occurrences of potential contacts to operators (see appendix D).

Seam Height Versus Random Variables

In comparing seam heights against boom direction, body part, and machine part (tables D–1 to D–3), the following relationships were identified. Regardless of seam height, contact incidents were always greater on the hand, always greater for the boom arm part of the machine, and always greater when the boom arm was moving up. The greatest number of contacts was always associated with the 60-in seam. The greatest number of contacts occurred for the 60-in seam with the boom moving up (46% of all contacts), the 60-in seam with contact on the hand (32% of all contacts), and the 60-in seam with contact made with the machine boom (47% of all contacts). The fewest number of contacts occurred for the 72-in seam with the boom moving down and the 45-in seam with contact made with the drill head. Zero contacts occurred with the operator's leg at a 45-in seam height and with the operator's head at a 72-in seam height.

Subject Versus Random Variables

In comparing subjects against boom arm direction, body part, and machine part (tables D–4 to D–6), the following relationships were identified. Regardless of subject size, contact incidents were always greater when the boom was moving up, always greater on the hand, and always greater for the boom part of the machine. The greatest number of contacts was always associated with the 25th-percentile size, and the fewest number of contacts always occurred with the 92nd-percentile size. The greatest number of contacts occurred for the 25th-percentile size with the boom moving up (29% of all contacts), occurred on the hand (27% of all contacts), and involved the machine boom (31% of all contacts). The fewest number of contacts occurred for the 92nd-percentile size with the boom moving down, occurred on the arm, and involved the drill head.

Work Posture Versus Random Variables

Analysts identified several relationships when comparing work posture against boom direction, body part, and machine part (see tables D–7 to D–9). Regardless of posture, contact incidents were always greater when the boom was moving up, always greater on the hand, and always greater for the boom part of the machine. The greatest number of contacts occurred for the both-knee work posture with the boom moving up (27% of all contacts), the right-knee posture with contact made with the hand (18% of all contacts), and the both-knee posture with contact made with the machine boom (25% of all contacts). The fewest number of contacts occurred for the standing posture with the boom moving down and for the standing posture with contact made with the drill head. Zero contacts occurred for the cases involving the operator's head in the right-knee, left-knee, and standing work postures and for those involving the operator's leg in the both-knee posture.

Drilling Behavior Versus Random Variables

Analysts identified several relationships when comparing drilling behavior against boom direction, body part, and machine part (see tables D–10 to D–12). Regardless of drilling behavior, contact incidents were always greater when the boom was moving up, always greater on the hand, and always greater for the boom part of the machine. The greatest number of contacts occurred for the hand-on-boom behavior with the boom moving up (42% of all contacts), occurred on the hand (41% of all contacts), and involved the machine boom (45% of all contacts). The fewest number of contacts occurred for the hand-on-drill-steel behavior with the boom moving down, hand-on-drill-steel behavior with contact on the arm, and hand-on-drill-steel-behavior involving the drill head part of the machine.

Bolting Behavior Versus Random Variables

Analysts identified several relationships when comparing bolting behavior against boom direction, body part, and machine part (see tables D–13 to D–15). Regardless of bolting behavior, contact incidents were always greater when the boom was moving up, always greater on the hand, and always greater for the boom part of the machine. The greatest number of contacts occurred for the hand-on-boom behavior with the boom moving up (26% of all contacts), occurred on the hand (27% of all contacts), and involved the machine boom (32% of all contacts). The fewest number of contacts occurred for the hand-on-bolt behavior with the boom moving down, the hand-on-boom-then-bolt behavior with contact on the arm, and the hand-on-bolt behavior with contact made with the drill head.

Boom Speed Versus Fixed, Conditional, and Random Variables

Analysts identified several relationships when comparing boom speed against boom direction, body part, and machine part (table D–16 to D–18). Regardless of boom speed, contact incidents were always greater when the boom was moving up, always greater on the hand, and always greater for the boom part of the machine. The greatest number of contacts occurred at the 16 in/sec speed for the following: boom moving up (17% of all contacts), hand part of the body (16% of all contacts), and the boom part of the machine (18% of all contacts). The fewest number of contacts occurred for the 10-in/sec speed with the boom moving down, the 7-in/sec speed involving contact with the arm, and the 22-in/sec speed involving contact with the drill head.

Analysts identified several relationships when comparing boom speed against work posture, subject, drilling behavior, bolting behavior, and seam height (tables D–19 to D–23). For all boom speeds, the work posture on both knees had the greatest number of contacts and the standing posture had the fewest number of contacts. The greatest number of contacts occurred for the 16-in/sec speed with the work posture on both knees; the fewest number of contacts occurred for the 22-in/sec speed while standing. Regardless of boom speed, the 25th-percentile sizes had the greatest number of contacts while, regardless of speed, the 92nd-percentile size had the fewest number of contacts. The greatest number of contacts occurred for the 13-in/sec speed at the 25th-percentile size. The fewest number of contacts occurred for the 10-in/sec speed at the 92nd-percentile size. Regardless of boom speed, the 60-in seam height had the greatest number of contacts. The 72-in seam had

the fewest number of contacts for all speeds except 10 in/sec, where the 45-in seam had the fewest. The greatest number of contacts was associated with the 16 in/sec speed at the 60-in seam height. The fewest number of contacts was for the 10-in/sec speed at the 45-in seam height. Regardless of boom speed, the hand-on-boom drilling behavior had the most contacts and, regardless of speed, the hand-on-boom bolting behavior had the most contacts. Regardless of speed, the hand-on-drill-steel drilling behavior had the fewest number of contacts and, regardless of speed, the hand-on-bolt bolting behavior had the fewest number of contacts. For the drilling behaviors, the greatest number of contacts was for 13 in/sec and hand on the boom; the fewest number of contacts was for 13 in/sec and hand on the drill steel. For the bolting behaviors, the greatest number of contacts was for 13 in/sec and hand on the boom; the fewest was for 10 in/sec and hand on the bolt.

Summary

The frequency-fixed variable analyses showed the following:
- The faster boom speeds of 16 and 22 in/sec combined accounted for the greatest number of contacts (43% of the total).
- The seam height of 60 in had the most contacts, with 59% of the total number of contacts and 25% of the avoid incidents.
- A work posture on both knees had the greatest number of contact incidents compared to other postures (32% of the total contacts).
- The 25th-percentile individual had slightly more contact incidents than the other size individuals.

The frequency-conditional variable analyses showed the following:
- 42% of all contacts occurred for the hand-on-boom behavior when the boom was moving up.
- 41% of all contacts occurred for the hand-on-boom behavior with contact made with the hand.
- 45% of all contacts occurred for the hand-on-boom behavior with contact made with the machine boom.

The frequency-random variable analyses showed the following:
- The hand was the closest body part to the moving boom arm and was involved in 67% of all contact incidents.
- The boom was the closest moving machine part to the operator and accounted for 80% of all contacts.
- Regardless of other variables, contact incidents were always greater when the boom was moving up.

The cross-tabulation/fixed-variable analyses showed the following:
- Regardless of boom speed, 92nd-percentile-sized operators experienced fewer contacts than other operator sizes.
- Regardless of boom speed, 25th-percentile-sized operators experienced more contacts than other operator sizes.

The cross-tabulation/fixed-random-variable analyses showed the following:

- 46% of all contacts occurred in the 60-in seam with the boom moving up.
- 47% of all contacts occurred in the 60-in seam and involved the machine boom.

LOGISTIC REGRESSION ANALYSIS

Method

An initial approach to the modeling of the roof bolter simulation data used logistic regression analysis. This statistical procedure is often used to investigate the relationship between a binary or dichotomous response (outcome variable) and a set of predictor variables (or covariates). For a binary response model, the response, Y, can take on one of two possible values, denoted for convenience by 1 or 0.

$$\text{logit}(p) \quad \log\left(\frac{p}{1-p}\right) = \alpha + \beta' x \quad (1)$$

where   x is a vector of explanatory variables,

$p = \Pr(Y = 1 \mid x)$,

α is the intercept parameter,

and β' is the vector of slope parameters.

Odds ratio (OR) estimates are computed from the parameter estimates. The OR is defined as the ratio of the odds for those with the response factor variable ($x = 1$) to the odds for those without the response factor variable ($x = 0$). The OR is obtained by exponentiation of the value of the parameter associated with the response factor. It indicates how the odds of an event change as, for example, a dichotomous response factor changes from 0 to 1. For instance, an OR of 2 means that the odds of an event when the response factor variable $x = 1$ are twice the odds of an event when $x = 0$. The linear logistic regression models in this study were fit by the method of maximum likelihood. In a very general sense, the method of maximum likelihood estimation yields values for the unknown model parameters, which maximizes the probability of obtaining the observed set of data.

For the roof bolter simulation data, the outcome contact variable was coded as "contact" ($Y = 1$) versus "avoid + no contact" ($Y = 0$). The predictor variables or covariates considered in this analysis were restricted to only those that remained static during a simulation execution. These included (1) seam height, (2) boom speed, (3) anthropometry, (4) work posture, and (5) a work posture/seam height combination. Work posture/seam height combination was used because the higher seam height used only one posture—standing. The logistic

regression analysis modeled the probability of a "contact" as a function of this set of covariates [$\Pr(Y = 1 \mid x)$]. The analysis included 5,250 simulation executions, and 52% of the simulations exhibited a contact between the boom and the operator. All models used data generated for an operator with slow reaction time in order to be consistent with the other analytical techniques used in this report.

Initially, researchers produced univariate logistic regression models (models with only one predictor variable or covariate). A final main effects multivariate model that included all of the covariates tested in the univariate models was generated. The method of reference cell coding was used for all of the covariates (SAS version 8.0). A covariate was considered to be significantly related to the outcome when the p-value of the Wald test was <0.05. All models had a statistically significant main effect for the covariate(s). This analysis investigated no interactions terms. R^2 value, based on the likelihood ratio chi-square for testing the null hypothesis that all the coefficients are zero, was calculated for all of the models. This R^2 is a generalized coefficient of determination that measures predictive power (it cannot be interpreted as a proportion of variance explained by the covariates). The results of the logistic regression analysis are presented in appendix E.

Results

Model 1

For this model, the covariate under consideration was seam height. The reference group was seam height equal to 45 in. For 60 in compared to 45 in, the likelihood of a contact was almost seven times greater (OR = 6.96). For 72 in compared to 45 in, the likelihood of a contact was six times greater (OR = 6.33). The R^2 was equal to 0.24, which is the largest value shown for any of the univariate models. Thus, for these logistic regression models, seam height is the most important predictor of the probability of a contact.

Model 2

The predictor variable in this model was boom speed. A boom speed of 7 in/sec was the reference level. The contact difference between 10 in/sec and the reference group was less likelihood of a contact. ORs of approximately 1.35 and 1.19 were found for 16 and 22 in/sec, respectively, compared to 7 in/sec. There was no significant effect found at 13 in/sec.

Model 3

Anthropometry was the covariate entered in this model. A virtual human model that represented an operator conforming to the 55th percentile was chosen as the reference group. At the 25th percentile, an operator would be 1.65 times more likely to be contacted, whereas at the 92nd percentile an operator would be less likely to be contacted (OR = 0.69).

Model 4

In this model, the predictor variable was work posture, with standing being the reference level. Being on the right knee, the left knee, or both knees, an operator would be less likely to be contacted (OR = 0.36, 0.35, and 0.60, respectively).

Model 5

This model represented a multivariate model. A multivariate analysis is a more comprehensive modeling of the data. In a multivariate logistic regression model, each estimated coefficient provides an estimate of the log odds adjusting for all other variables included in the model. For this model, a problem occurred when seam height and anthropometry were included simultaneously. A linear combination occurred because the cells were empty for standing in 45- and 60-in seam heights and kneeling in 72-in seam heights. To handle this situation, a new variable was created that combined both seam height and work posture. "Standing/72 in" was considered the reference level, with the other categories being "right knee/45 in," "right knee/60 in," "left knee/45 in," "left knee/60 in," "both knees/45 in," and "both knees/60 in". For this new variable, the only OR that showed significant contact compared to "standing/72 in" was "both knees/60 in" (OR = 2.05). In this model, a 25th-percentile operator would be about two times more likely (OR = 1.93) to be contacted compared to the 55th-percentile reference level. Boom speeds of 16 and 22 in/sec were approximately 1.5 and 1.26 times more likely, respectively, of involving a contact compared to 7 in/sec.

In order to incorporate the predictor variables that were dynamic over the course of a simulation execution, it was necessary to use a modeling approach that took into account the element of time. Survival analysis (e.g., Cox regression) was the next step used for the modeling of the roof bolter simulation data.

Summary

• Compared to seam height of 45 in, the likelihood of a contact was nearly seven times greater in a seam height of 60 in and six times greater in a seam height of 72 in.

• The odds of a contact between a boom speed of 13 in/sec and 7 in/sec, the reference group, were not significant.

• ORs of approximately 1.35 and 1.19 were found for boom speeds of 16 and 22 in/sec, respectively, compared to 7 in/sec.

• A 25th-percentile operator is 1.65 times more likely to be contacted than a 55th-percentile operator. A 92nd-percentile operator is less likely to be contacted (OR = 0.69) than a 55th-percentile operator.

• Comparing work postures/seam heights, the operator has about the same likelihood of a contact when on the right knee, left knee, or both knees.

• For the multivariate model (comparing standing posture, 7 in/sec boom speed, and 55th-percentile operator), significantly higher ORs were found: 2.05 for "both knees/60 in," 1.5 for 16 in/sec and 1.26 for 22 in/sec, and 1.93 for the 25th-percentile operator.

SURVIVAL ANALYSIS

The following describes the results of a survival analysis on the simulations presented in this report. Some of the information presented regarding the methods and results of the survival analysis are somewhat technical. However, a summary at the end of this section describes the major findings of the survival analysis for those not interested in the technical aspects of the analysis.

Method

Variables Investigated

Several variables believed to be important in influencing whether and when a contact might occur were investigated. These include boom speed, drilling and bolting behaviors, boom direction (up or down), work posture/seam height combinations (e.g., worker on right knee in 45-in seam), operator location, and anthropometry (worker size). The dependent (or the outcome) variable was the time to an event (i.e., boom making contact with the worker) occurring.

Except for operator location, which was entered as a continuous variable, all variables in the model were entered as dummy variables using a referent (or comparison) condition against which all other levels of the variable were judged. The following list identifies the referent conditions for all independent variables for which dummy coding were used.

• Boom speed: 7 in/sec
• Drilling behavior: hand not touching boom or drill steel
• Bolting behavior: hand not touching boom or bolt
• Work posture/seam height combination: standing in 72-in seam
• Anthropometry: 25th-percentile worker
• Boom direction: boom not moving upwards
• Operator location: distance from operator's back to boom is 23 in

Data

Researchers examined 5,250 cases involving possible contact between the boom arm and the operator. A number of cases involved no contact between the operator and the boom while the boom was not moving. As a result, the survival analysis comprised 3,517 cases. Of this total, 2,750 cases involved unintentional contact with a moving boom arm (considered an "event" in the survival analysis). The balance (767 cases) consisted of censored observations or cases where unintentional contact between the boom arm and operator occurred throughout the simulation execution.

Survival Analysis

A Cox regression model (time-to-event regression analysis) was conducted to evaluate the factors influencing the time when contact was made to the worker. Table 11 shows the hypothesized time-to-event regression model. Analysts used a forward selection procedure in developing the model. In each step, variables were selected for inclusion on the basis of the Akaike Information Criterion (AIC), i.e., the model whose variable resulted in the lowest AIC was selected at each successive step of the model-building process. The model-building process ceased when the lowest AIC for a step was greater than the lowest AIC obtained in the previous step.

A primary assumption of the time-to-event regression model was that the hazard proportions associated with the model's variable comparisons did not differ significantly with respect to time during the period of analysis. This assumption was checked for all variables at the univariate stage of the model-building process. If the assumption was not tenable, the interaction between the variable and the natural logarithm of time was included in the model whenever that variable was entered into the regression models. A final check of the proportional hazards assumption was performed once the final model was determined.

Probabilities that risk ratios were significantly different from 1 were calculated using the Wald statistic for covariates with one degree of freedom. Probabilities for variables with multiple degrees of freedom were obtained by subtracting the log likelihood for the reduced model from the full model and obtaining a chi-square with the appropriate degrees of freedom. Alpha levels were set at 0.05 for all cases. Results for each step of the survival analysis are presented in appendix F.

Results

Results of Forward Selection Process

Variables entered earlier in the model-building process are considered more influential for predicting the time-to-event (contacts) than those entered later. The following list shows the order in which variables were entered into the model:

1. Boom speed
2. Boom direction
3. Drilling behavior
4. Work posture/seam height combination
5. Bolting behavior
6. Anthropometry (operator percentile)
7. Operator location

Tables F–1 to F–7 contain results of the analyses in the development of the main effects model. These tables reveal that the first five variables included in the model violated the proportional hazards assumption. This indicates that the hazard associated with a contact occurring was not constant over the period of the analysis, but that the hazard changed over time.

Thus, in the final model (table F–8), these variables included interaction terms with the natural logarithm of time to properly assess the associated risks throughout the period of the simulation.

Risk Model

Based on the results of the forward selection Cox regression analyses, a main effects risk model was developed (table 12). The coefficients in this model helped to evaluate the relative risk of experiencing a contact at different points during the simulation executions and showed the degree of influence for each variable in the model while controlling for the effects of all other covariates. For example, if one wanted to know the relative risk of a contact for a worker bolting with the boom moving up at 16 in/sec at time 25 (compared to reference conditions), one would simply insert a "1" for each term containing a z_2 and z_7, a "25" for each term with ln (time) included, and a "0" for all other variables. The result would be that such a worker would have a chance of experiencing a contact that was 33.25 times the referent condition.

Table 13 shows the instantaneous relative risk of experiencing a contact for all model variables at different times in the simulation process. Each estimate of risk of experiencing a contact represents the increase (or decrease) in the chance of a contact occurring at a particular time assuming that the specified variable is present and that the influencing factor is judged against the referent condition. The following sections detail the implications of the relative risk model in terms of the independent variables examined.

Boom Speed

Boom speed was the most influential variable in terms of explaining the time to an event (contact) occurring. Increases in boom speed resulted in increased chance of a contact throughout the period of the simulation. Thus, based on the data collected in this simulation analysis, boom speeds greater than 13 in/sec result in a substantial increase in chance that the roof bolter operator would be contacted, while speeds less than or equal to 13 in/sec are associated with a more modest hazard level.

Boom Direction

Relative risk of being contacted for the boom moving in an upward direction (compared to downward or no movement) were greatest at the beginning of the task and decreased with time. Early in the task, upward movement of the boom resulted in a threefold increase in the chance of a contact. At the midpoint of the simulation (time = 25), the relative chance was still more than twice the referent condition. This change in the hazard reflects the fact that conditions where the boom is moving upward occur earlier, on average, than situations where the boom is moving downward. Thus, the risk of being contacted associated with upward boom movement tend to be seen earlier in the simulation rather than later. In general, chances of a contact were greater for upward compared to downward boom movement.

Drilling Behavior

Analysts found hand placements when drilling to result in significant increases in the chance of a contact occurring early in the simulation, with decreasing chances observed as the simulation time increased. This chance of being contacted profile reflects the fact that the drilling phase of roof bolting occurs early in the task, and chance of a contact associated with this activity would be seen early in the simulation. Having the hand on the drill steel then the boom resulted in the greatest increase in chances of being contacted compared with the hand being on neither the drill steel nor the boom. Having the hand only on the boom was associated with an only slightly less chance of a contact than having the hand on the drill steel then boom, but a greater chance than when having the hand on the drill steel.

Table 11. Hypothesized time-to-event regression model

$$h(t \mid z) = h_0(t \mid z)\exp\left(\begin{array}{l}\beta_{\overline{1}}z_1 + \beta_{\overline{2}}z_2 + \beta_{\overline{3}}z_3 + \beta_{\overline{4}}z_4 + \beta_{\overline{5}}z_5 + \beta_{\overline{6}}z_6 + \beta_{\overline{7}}z_7 + \beta_{\overline{8}}z_8 + \beta_{\overline{9}}z_9 + \beta_{\overline{10}}z_{10} + \beta_{\overline{11}}z_{11} \\ \pm \beta_{\overline{12}}z_{12} + \beta_{\overline{13}}z_{13} + \beta_{\overline{14}}z_{14} + \beta_{\overline{15}}z_{15} + \beta_{\overline{16}}z_{16} + \beta_{\overline{17}}z_{17} + \beta_{\overline{18}}z_{18} + \beta_{\overline{19}}z_{19} + \beta_{\overline{20}}z_{20}\end{array}\right) =$$

β_k = coefficients for variables used in the model;
z_1 = boom speed 10 in/sec;
z_2 = boom speed 13 in/sec;
z_3 = boom speed 16 in/sec;
z_4 = boom speed 22 in/sec;
z_5 = boom moving upwards;
z_6 = drilling behavior: hand on drill steel;
z_7 = drilling behavior: hand on boom;
z_8 = drilling behavior: hand on drill steel then on boom;
z_9 = posture/seam: right knee/45 in;
z_{10} = posture/seam: right knee/60 in;

z_{11} = posture/seam: left knee/45 in;
z_{12} = posture/seam: left knee/60 in;
z_{13} = posture/seam: both knees/45 in;
z_{14} = posture/seam: both knees/60 in;
z_{15} = bolting behavior: hand on bolt;
z_{16} = bolting behavior: hand on boom;
z_{17} = bolting behavior: hand on bolt then on boom;
z_{18} = 55th-percentile worker;
z_{19} = 95th-percentile worker; and
z_{20} = operator location (in).

Table 12. Main effects risk model

$$h(t \mid z) \quad h_0(t \mid z)\exp(-2.300 * z_1 + 1.173 * z_1 * \ln(time) - 3.698 * z_2 + 1.971 * z_2 * \ln(time) - 3.890 * z_3 +$$
$$2.299 * z_3 * \ln(time) - 4.234 * z_4 + 2.649 * z_4 * \ln(time) + 2.995 * z_5 - 0.668 * z_5 * \ln(time) + 3.906 * z_6 -$$
$$1.142 * z_6 * \ln(time) + 4.978 * z_7 - 1.428 * z_7 * \ln(time) - 5.282 * z_8 - 1.465 * z_8 * \ln(time) - 9.236 * z_9 +$$
$$3.927 * z_9 * \ln(time) - 6.049 * z_{10} + 2.291 * z_{10} * \ln(time) - 9.470 * z_{11} + 3.959 * z_{11} * \ln(time) - 6.002 * z_{12} +$$
$$2.274 * z_{12} * \ln(time) - 9.014 * z_{13} + 3.743 * z_{13} * \ln(time) - 2.539 * z_{14} + 1.137 * z_{14} * \ln(time) + 0.675 * z_{15} -$$
$$0.341 * \ln(time) + 0.250 * z_{16} - 0.230 * z_{16} * \ln(time) + 0.241 * z_{17} - 0.268 * z_{17} * \ln(time) + 0.047 * z_{18} +$$
$$0.243 * z_{19} - 0.170 * z_{20})$$

z_1 = boom speed 10 in/sec;
z_2 = boom speed 13 in/sec;
z_3 = boom speed 16 in/sec;
z_4 = boom speed 22 in/sec;
z_5 = boom moving upwards;
z_6 = drilling behavior: hand on drill steel;
z_7 = drilling behavior: hand on boom;
z_8 = drilling behavior: hand on drill steel then on boom;
z_9 = posture/seam: right knee/45 in;
z_{10} = posture/seam: right knee/60 in;

z_{11} = posture/seam: left knee/45 in;
z_{12} = posture/seam: left knee/60 in;
z_{13} = posture/seam: both knees/45 in;
z_{14} = posture/seam: both knees/60 in;
z_{15} = bolting behavior: hand on bolt;
z_{16} = bolting behavior: hand on boom;
z_{17} = bolting behavior: hand on bolt then on boom;
z_{18} = 55th-percentile worker;
z_{19} = 95th-percentile worker; and
z_{20} = operator location (in).

Table 13. Instantaneous relative risk estimates at specified time for each variable

Variable	Time = 15	Time = 25	Time = 35	Time = 45
Boom speed, in/sec:				
10	2.40	4.37	6.49	8.72
13	5.15	14.10	27.37	44.92
16	10.34	33.45	72.49	129.20
22	18.89	73.14	178.38	347.11
Boom moving up	3.27	2.33	1.85	1.58
Drilling behavior:				
Hand on drill steel	2.25	1.26	0.86	0.64
Hand on boom	3.03	1.47	0.91	0.64
Hand on drill steel then on boom ...	3.73	1.77	1.07	0.75
Work posture/seam height:				
Right knee/45 in	4.05	30.10	112.80	302.63
Right knee/60 in	1.18	3.75	8.12	14.47
Left knee/45 in	3.48	26.40	100.02	270.52
Left knee/60 in	1.18	3.73	8.01	14.20
Both knees/45 in	3.08	20.77	73.22	187.60
Both knees/60 in	1.72	3.06	4.50	5.98
Bolting behavior:				
Hand on bolt	0.78	0.64	0.59	0.54
Hand on boom	0.70	0.62	0.56	0.54
Hand on bolt then on boom	0.62	0.54	0.48	0.46
Operator percentile:				
55th	1.05	1.05	1.05	1.05
92nd	1.29	1.29	1.29	1.29
Operator location, in	.017*OPLOC	.017*OPLOC	.017*OPLOC	.017*OPLOC

Work Posture/Seam Height Combinations

Table 13 shows a number of interesting relationships related to the effects of work posture and seam height. First, all restricted posture/seam combinations increase the chance of a contact to the worker (or decrease the time-to-event) compared to a standing posture in a 72-in seam. However, this effect is particularly pronounced in the 45-in seam, with very high chances of being contacted observed in this low seam height. These results clearly show the increased threat of contact to the operator as seam heights diminish. However, the kneeling postures used also seem to affect the time to an event occurring. Within each seam height, the greatest chance of a contact was associated with kneeling on the right knee. Kneeling on the left knee had a slightly less chance of a contact, while kneeling on both knees had the lowest chance. These findings indicate possible recommendation to change work posture that might significantly reduce the chance of workers making contact with the boom of the roof bolter machine.

Bolting Behavior

Coefficients for bolting behaviors were all less than 1, indicating a protective effect. This is because the bolting task is done late in the simulation. Any contact due to these bolting behaviors will happen relatively late in the simulation sequence, resulting in a longer time-to-event.

Anthropometry

Model coefficients suggest that larger (92nd-percentile) workers have about a 25% increased chance of experiencing a contact (or being contacted more quickly) compared to smaller (25th-percentile) workers. Average size workers (55th-percentile) enjoy an obvious reduction in the chance of making contact, about 5% lower than for small-size workers.

Operator Location

The negative coefficient for the operator location variable (a continuous variable) shows that the greater the distance between the operator and the boom, the less likely the operator will be to experience a contact (or the longer it will take for a contact to occur). Compared to the referent condition where the operator's back is 23 in from the boom, moving an additional 9 in away will reduce the relative risk by 31%. The maximum operator location distance studied, 38 in, reduced the relative risk by 50% compared to the referent. Although moving the operator farther away from the boom decreases the chance of a contact, it should be noted that this could also make the operator's job more difficult. For example, greater strength demands would be required to handle a bolt or drill steel farther from the body. However, this data analysis suggests that bolter operators should position themselves as far away from the boom as possible, and this will not compromise their ability to perform the bolting task.

Summary

One of the main interests in performing this survival analysis was to determine the impact of boom speed on the chance of experiencing a contact in these simulations of roof bolter activities. Results show that boom arm speed was the most influential factor in terms of affecting the chance of a contact occurring and the time at which such a contact might occur.

Moreover, results of this analysis show that there is a significant increase in the risk of being contacted at the two highest boom speeds, 16 and 22 in/sec, compared to the lower speeds (13 in/sec or less). The former were associated with a marked, and perhaps unacceptable, increase in the risk of being contacted, whereas the risk for the latter was much more modest. From the current analysis, one can conclude that boom speeds above 13 in/sec entail significant chance of being contacted. Speeds that are 13 in/sec or below result in a much lower exposure to being contacted, which represents a decrease in potential hazard.

Covariates such as operator work behaviors (placing the hand on the boom, drill steel, or bolt), work posture and seam height combinations, boom direction, operator location, and worker anthropometry were also significant factors in the time-to-event regression analysis. Workers were more likely to experience a contact when the boom was moving in an upward direction, especially early in the roof bolting task. Kneeling work postures generally resulted in increased risk of being contacted compared to standing in a 72-in seam. Kneeling on the right knee within each seam height entailed the greatest chance of a contact. Positioning of the workers farther from the boom resulted in a lower risk of being contacted; however, this could also impact the workers' ability to perform the roof bolting task. Larger workers were 25% more likely to make contact with the boom, whereas smaller workers were about 5% less likely to make contact. Drilling behaviors such as placing the hand on the boom or drill steel resulted in a greater chance of a contact, while bolting behaviors (occurring later in the bolting cycle) increased the time when the event occurred.

It should be noted that this survival analysis was developed using a main effects model only. It is possible that the factors examined in this report have interactive effects (for instance, boom speed could have more of an impact on the chance of being contacted when certain work postures are adopted). The large number of simulations, computational demands of running Cox regression models and of checking proportional hazard assumptions, and the large number of interactions (120) made analysis of these interactions impractical given the time constraints involved.

CONCLUSIONS

NIOSH researchers successfully developed a computer model that generates contact data by means of simulation while exercising the model with several variables associated with the machine and its operator, such as coal seam height, the operator's anthropometry, work posture and choice of risky behavior, and the machine's appendage velocity. The resulting simulation database contains 5,250 observations. The database represented the equivalence of actual field observations of roof bolting and corresponds to a work period of 12.15 eight-hour shifts.

Analysts used data only on the occurrences for the operator with slow reactions that included one incident per simulation execution (one run/one contact). Researchers on this project believe the use of such simulations, treated with statistical procedures such as frequency, cross-tabulation, logistic regression, and survival analysis, provide extremely useful tools to evaluate the hazards of tasks where it is not possible to perform experiments with human subjects. Results of this analysis could help in making recommendations that reduce the likelihood that roof bolter operators experience injuries due to contact with a moving boom.

Analysis shows that the reaction time of the operator did not significantly affect the outcome of the simulation. The number of contact incidents for an operator with slow reactions differed from those for an operator with fast reactions by less than 1% in both data sets. There was a reasonable difference in reaction times between fast and slow operators obtained from reaction time tests on our human subjects. As to the reason for the small difference in contacts, researchers speculate that in the boom speed range studied, if the operator with fast reactions could not get out of the path of the boom, the slower operator certainly would not either.

Results from frequency distribution analyses showed:

• The seam height of 60 in had the most contacts (59% of the total number of contacts), and the seam height of 45 in had 75% of the avoid incidents.

• The 25th-percentile individual had 7% more contacts than the 55th-percentile and 13% more than the 92nd-percentile.

• The one-knee work posture had 49% of the total number of contact incidents, the posture on both knees had 32%, and the standing posture had 19%.

• The faster boom speeds of 16 and 22 in/sec combined accounted for the greatest number of contacts (43% of the total).

• The hand-on-boom behavior for both drilling and bolting tasks accounted for most of the contacts.

• The boom-up direction had the most contacts (76% of the total number of contacts). The boom-down direction had 63% of the avoid incidents.

• The hand was the closest body part to the moving boom arm and was involved in 67% of all contacts. The leg was the second most contacted body part (15% of all contacts).

• The boom was the closest moving machine part to the operator, accounting for 80% of all contacts.

• Regardless of other variables, contact incidents were always greater when the boom was moving up, always greater on the hand, and always greater for the boom arm part of the machine. The reason why the subject experiences more contacts when the boom arm is moving up rather than down is that riskier behaviors occur during drilling and bolting, when the boom is ascending.

Results regarding boom speed from cross-tabulation analyses showed:

- Regardless of boom speed, the boom-up direction had more contacts than boom-down.
- The boom-up direction had most of its contacts at the two higher boom speeds: 22% at speed 16 in/sec and 21% at speed 22 in/sec.
- Regardless of boom speed, the operator's hand had more contacts than the other body parts.
- The hand had most of its contacts during speed 16 in/sec (24%) and 13 in/sec (21%).
- The boom arm had more contacts than the drill head and had most contacts during speeds 16 and 22 in/sec.
- The both-knee work posture had more contacts than the other postures and had most contacts (23%) during speed 16 in/sec.
- 25th-percentile operators had more contacts than other operator sizes and had most of their contacts (22%) during speed 13 in/sec.
- Regardless of boom speed, the hand-on-boom behavior during drilling and bolting tasks had more contacts than other work behaviors.
- Drilling tasks had most of their contacts (24%) during speed 13 in/sec. Bolting had most contacts (22%) during the same speed.
- The 60-in seam had more contacts than the other seam heights and had most of the contacts (22%) during speed 16 in/sec.

Logistic regression analyses showed:

- Compared to a seam height of 45 in, contacts occurred nearly seven times more often in a 60-in seam height and six times more often in a 72-in seam height.
- The odds of a contact between a boom speed of 13 and 7 in/sec, the reference group, were not significant.

- ORs of approximately 1.35 and 1.19 were found for 16 and 22 in/sec, respectively, compared to 7 in/sec.
- A 25th-percentile operator had a likelihood of making more contacts (1.65) than a 55th-percentile operator.
- A 92nd-percentile operator had a likelihood of making fewer contacts (0.69) than a 55th-percentile operator.
- Comparing work postures/seam heights, about the same likelihood of a contact occurred when the operator was on the right knee, left knee, or both knees.
- For the multivariate model (comparing standing posture, 7-in/sec boom speed, and 55th-percentile operator), significantly higher ORs were found: 2.05 for both knees/60 in, 1.5 for 16 in/sec and 1.26 for 22 in/sec, and 1.93 for the 25th-percentile operator.

Results of a survival analytic approach showed:

- Controlling the boom speed is the most important factor in determining the chance of an operator making contact.
- Boom speed was the most influential variable for explaining the time to an event (contact) occurring.
- Increases in boom speed resulted in increased chance of a contact throughout the period of the simulation.
- The chance of being contacted at the higher boom speeds (16 and 22 in/sec) was generally two to four times greater than at 13 in/sec and four to eight times greater than at 10 in/sec.
- A boom arm speed greater than 16 in/sec resulted in a substantial increase in the chance of the boom making contact with the roof bolter operator.
- Boom speeds less than or equal to 13 in/sec resulted in a smaller chance of being contacted, which represents a decrease in potential hazard.

OTHER RESEARCH CONSIDERATIONS

The process of performing 5,250 simulations and subsequent analyses required a considerable effort. Automating the simulation software and integrating data management with data analysis can enhance the virtual-reality simulation method. Software automation can decrease the time required to produce simulations and permit more time for data analysis. The integration of data management and data analysis can increase efficiency and permit an extensive examination of available information. For instance, a central database could streamline software automation by providing a queue of requested simulations, real-time monitoring of active simulations, and archived data from completed simulations. Simple data analysis interfaces could query data directly from the database and allow researchers to update calculations as data become available. In addition, enhanced data analysis interfaces would trigger calculations within the database or initiate iterative computations on a remote system; this would increase the efficiency of repetitive analyses and permit an unparalleled degree of exploratory data analysis. Individual researchers could use interfaces tailored to their specific roles. Virtual-reality simulations provide a wealth of information that is unavailable through conventional investigations. These automation, data management, and data analysis enhancements could efficiently represent this information and allow investigators to draw insightful conclusions regarding health and safety issues.

Analysts answered this study's question concerning boom speed by using the most appropriate statistical techniques available. Other factors such as drilling behavior, bolting behavior, boom direction, work posture/seam height combination, operator location, and anthropometry showed significant influence on the chance of an operator making contact. Using analytical techniques, an examination of the database would uncover significant interactions between these factors should they exist.

Researchers recommended a study to increase the safety for bolting machine operators during lateral boom swing operations.

This research has been approved and is currently underway. Boom swing usually occurs when the operator is repositioning the boom arm to a new bolt insertion location. It requires that the operator properly actuate the right control(s) and then reposition his/her body in coordination with the moving boom arm. In low seam heights, operators may perform boom swings from kneeling positions, which hinders their ability to avoid contact with the boom arm. Observation of boom swing shows that even experienced operators have a tendency to actuate the boom swing control in the direction opposite from what is intended. The fundamental issue is which boom swing speed(s) maximize the operators' chances of escaping injuries while still allowing the operators to perform bolting functions effectively. Like the vertical boom arm study, this work will use primarily motion capture and computer simulation/modeling technologies to evaluate human motions while operating a bolting machine in various postures. Expected outcomes include lateral boom swing velocities, possible control, and procedural modifications to minimize inadvertent control actuation.

ACKNOWLEDGMENTS

The authors gratefully acknowledge the following colleagues at the NIOSH Pittsburgh Research Laboratory: Joseph P. DuCarme, Mary Ellen Nelson, Albert H. Cook, George F. Fischer, Albert L. Brautigam provided technical expertise in the design and fabrication of the roof bolter mockup and platform, and the associated electrical and hydraulic control systems. E. William Rossi provided technical support in operating the motion tracking and data collection system. Mary Ellen Nelson, Albert H. Cook, and Mary Ann Rossi assisted in the lab human subject tests.

REFERENCES

Ambrose DH [2000]. A simulation approach analyzing random motion events between a machine and its operator. Warrendale, PA: Society of Automotive Engineers, Inc., technical paper 2000 01 2160, pp. 1 11.

Ambrose DH [2001]. Random motion capture model for studying events between a machine and its operator. In: Proceedings of the Advanced Simulation Technologies Conference (Seattle, WA, April 22 26, 2001). San Diego, CA: Society for Computer Simulation International, pp. 127 134.

Ambrose DH [2004]. Developing random virtual human motions and risky work behaviors for studying anthropotechnical systems. Pittsburgh, PA: U.S. Department of Health and Human Services, Public Health Service, Centers for Disease Control and Prevention, National Institute for Occupational Safety and Health, DHHS (NIOSH) Publication No. 2004 130, IC 9468.

Bartels JR, Ambrose DH, Wang RC [2001]. Verification and validation of roof bolter simulation models for studying events between a machine and its operator. Warrendale, PA: Society of Automotive Engineers, Inc., technical paper 2001 01 2088, pp. 1 14.

Bartels JR, Kwitowski AJ, Ambrose DH [2003]. Verification of a roof bolter simulation model. Warrendale, PA: Society of Automotive Engineers, Inc., technical paper 2003 01 2217, pp. 1 7.

Etherton J [1987]. System considerations on robot end effector speed as a risk factor during robot maintenance. In: Proceedings of the Eighth International System Safety Conference (New Orleans, LA). Unionville, VA: System Safety Society, pp. 434 437.

Helander MG, Karwan MH, Etherton J [1987]. A model of human reaction time to dangerous robot arm movements. In: Proceedings of the 31st Annual Meeting of the Human Factors Society. Santa Monica, CA: Human Factors Society, pp. 191 195.

Humantech, Inc. [2003]. Ergonomic design guidelines for engineers. Ann Arbor, MI: Humantech, Inc.

Karwowski W, Parsaei HR, Soundararajan A, Pongpatanasuegsa N [1992]. Estimation of safe distance from the robot arm as a guide for limiting slow speed of robot motions. In: Proceedings of the 36th Annual Meeting of the Human Factors and Ergonomics Society. Santa Monica, CA: Human Factors and Ergonomics Society, pp. 992 996.

Klishis MJ, Althous RC, Layne LA, Lies GM [1993a]. Coal mine injury analysis: a model for reduction through training. Morgantown, WV: West Virginia University, Mining Extension Service.

Klishis MJ, Althous RC, Stobbe TJ, Plummer RW, Grayson RL, Layne LA, et al. [1993b]. Coal mine injury analysis: a model for reduction through training. Vol. 8: Accident risk during the roof bolting cycle: analysis of problems and potential solutions, Morgantown, WV: West Virginia University. Mining Extension Service.

Kobrick JL [1965]. Effects of physical location of visual stimuli on intentional response time. J Eng Psychol 4(1):1 8.

MSHA [1994]. Coal mine safety and health roof bolting machine committee: report of findings, July 8, 1994. Arlington, VA: U.S. Department of Labor, Mine Safety and Health Administration, Coal Mine Safety and Health, Safety Division, pp. 1 28.

OSHA [1987]. Guidelines for robotic safety. OSHA directive STD 01 12 002 (instruction pub 8 1.3). Washington, DC: U.S. Department of Labor, Occupational Safety and Health Administration, Office of Science and Technology Assessment, September 21.

Turin FC, et al. [1995]. Human factors analysis of roof bolting hazards in underground coal mines. Pittsburgh, PA: U.S. Department of the Interior, Bureau of Mines, RI 9568. NTIS No. PB 95 274411.

U.S. Department of Energy [1998]. Department of Energy (DOE) OSH technical reference. Chapter 1 industrial robots; part 4 work practices; 4.1 safeguarding methods. [http://www.eh.doe.gov/docs/osh_tr/ch14.html]. Date accessed: January 2005.

Volberg O, Ambrose DH [2002]. Motion editing and reuse techniques and their role in studying events between a machine and its operator. In: Proceedings of the Society of Computer Simulation International Advanced Simulation Technologies Conference (San Diego, CA, April 14 18). Vol. 34, No. 4. San Diego, CA: Society of Computer Simulation International, pp. 181 186.

Welford AT, Brebner JMT [1980]. Reaction times. New York: Academic Press, pp. 117 123.

APPENDIX A.–FREQUENCY OF INCIDENTS

Figure A 1. Incidents by seam height.

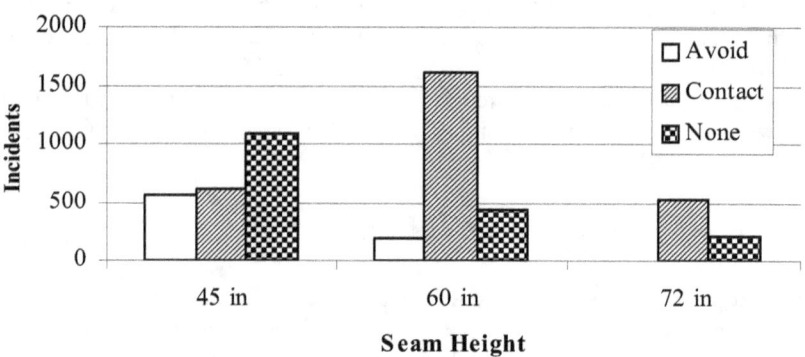

Table A 1. Incidents by seam height

Seam height, in	Avoid	Contact	None	Total
45	564	606	1,080	2,250
60	185	1,619	446	2,250
72	6	525	219	750
Total	755	2,750	1,745	5,250

Figure A 2. Incidents by operator percentile.

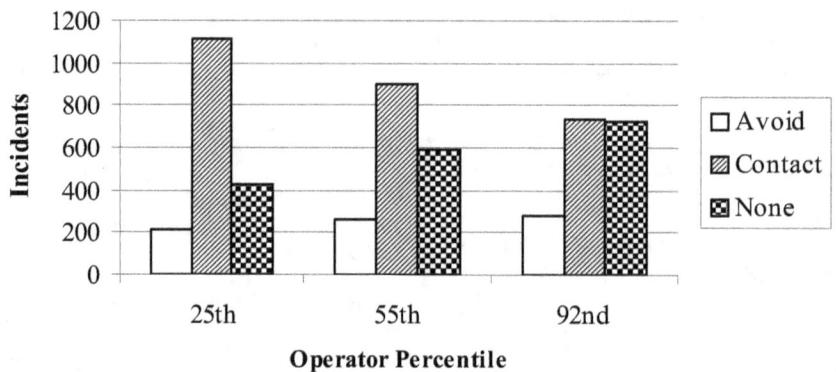

Table A 2. Incidents by operator percentile

Operator percentile	Avoid	Contact	None	Total
25th	211	1,113	426	1,750
55th	259	900	592	1,751
92nd	285	737	727	1,749
Total	755	2,750	1,745	5,250

Figure A 3.   Incidents by work posture.

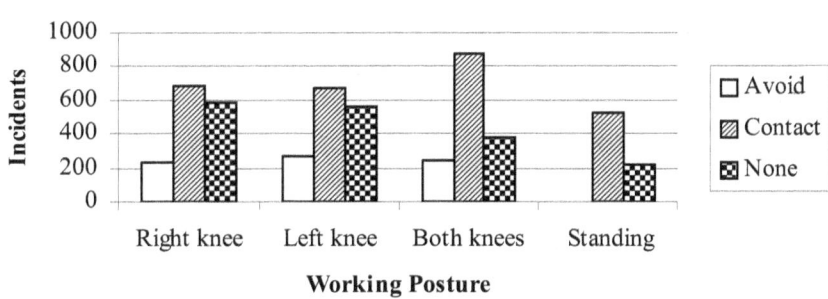

Table A 3.   Incidents by work posture

Work posture	Avoid	Contact	None	Total
Right knee	237	682	581	1,500
Left knee	268	669	563	1,500
Both knees	244	874	382	1,500
Standing	6	525	219	750
Total	755	2,750	1,745	5,250

Figure A 4.   Incidents by boom speed.

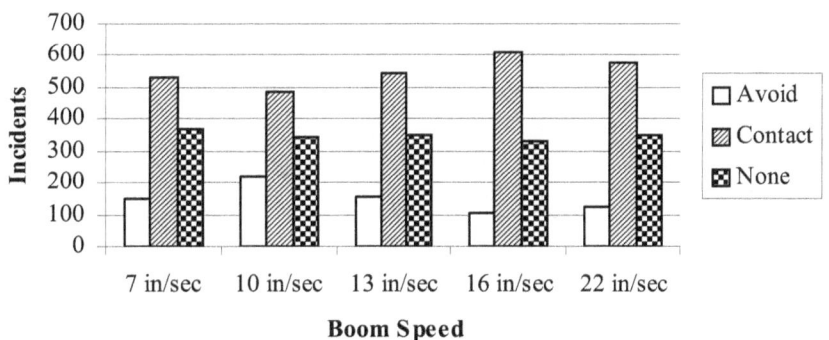

Table A 4.   Incidents by boom speed

Boom speed, in/sec	Avoid	Contact	None	Total
7	147	533	370	1,050
10	223	486	341	1,050
13	157	542	351	1,050
16	106	611	333	1,050
22	122	578	350	1,050
Total	755	2,750	1,745	5,250

Figure A 5. Incidents by drilling behavior.

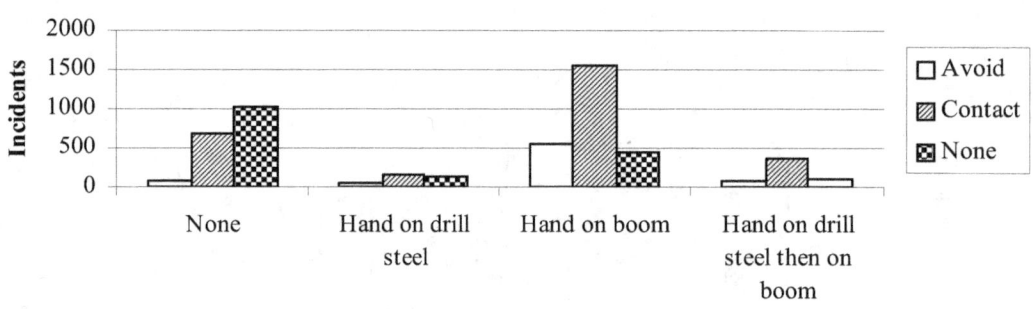

Drilling Behavior

Table A 5. Incidents by drilling behavior

Drilling behavior	Avoid	Contact	None	Total
None	68	673	1,030	1,771
Hand on drill steel	42	168	142	352
Hand on boom	555	1,541	458	2,554
Hand on drill steel then on boom	90	368	115	573
Total	755	2,750	1,745	5,250

Figure A 6. Incidents by bolting behavior.

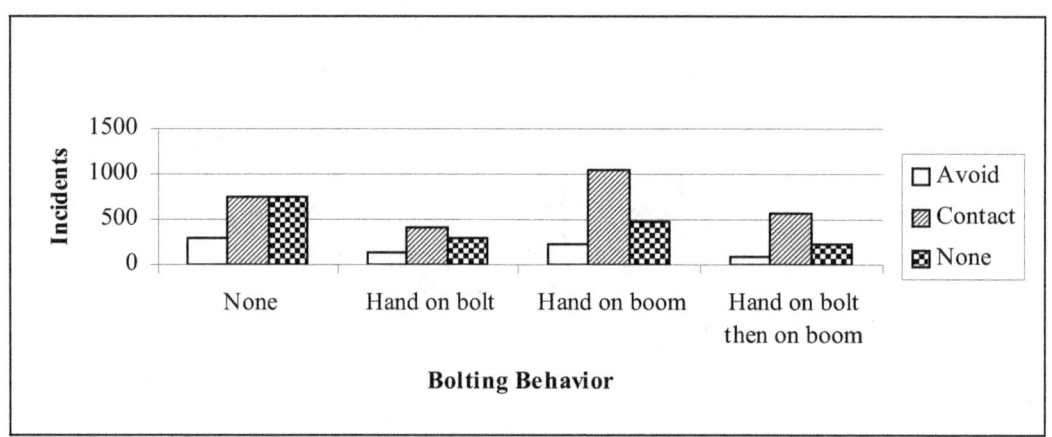

Bolting Behavior

Table A 6. Incidents by bolting behavior

Bolting behavior	Avoid	Contact	None	Total
None	287	748	756	1,791
Hand on bolt	146	402	289	837
Hand on boom	220	1,042	468	1,730
Hand on bolt then on boom	102	558	232	892
Total	755	2,750	1,745	5,250

Figure A 7. Incidents by boom direction.

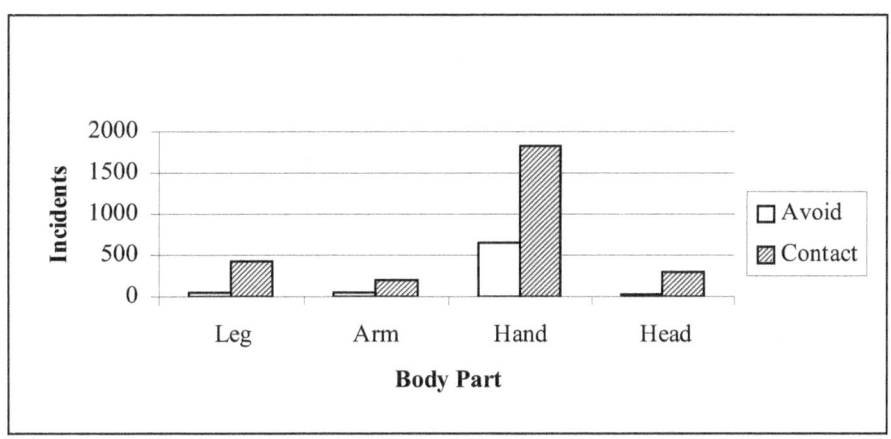

Table A 7. Incidents by boom direction

Boom direction	Avoid	Contact	Total
Down	472	671	1,143
Up	283	2,079	2,362
Total	755	2,750	3,505

Figure A 8. Incidents by body part.

Table A 8. Incidents by body part

Body part	Avoid	Contact	Total
Leg	51	419	470
Arm	38	201	239
Hand	638	1,835	2,473
Head	28	295	323
Total	755	2,750	3,505

Figure A 9. Incidents by machine part.

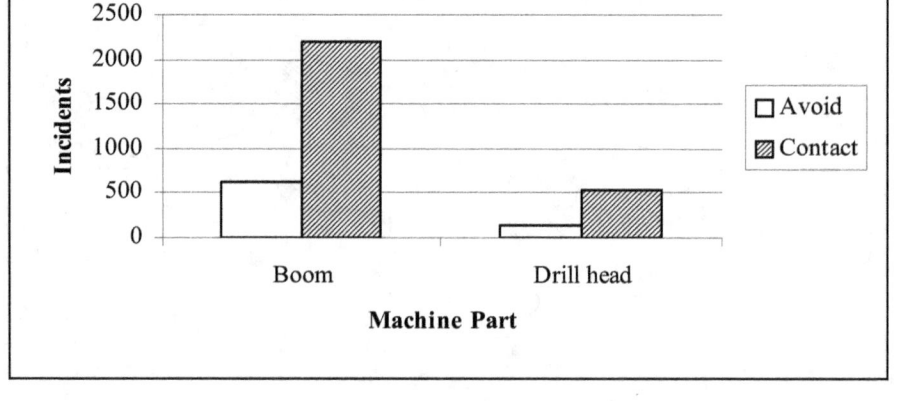

Table A 9. Incidents by machine part

Machine part	Avoid	Contact	Total
Boom	622	2,209	2,831
Drill head	133	541	674
Total	755	2,750	3,505

APPENDIX B.–FREQUENCY BY OPERATOR LOCATION

Figure B 1.   Incidents by operator location.

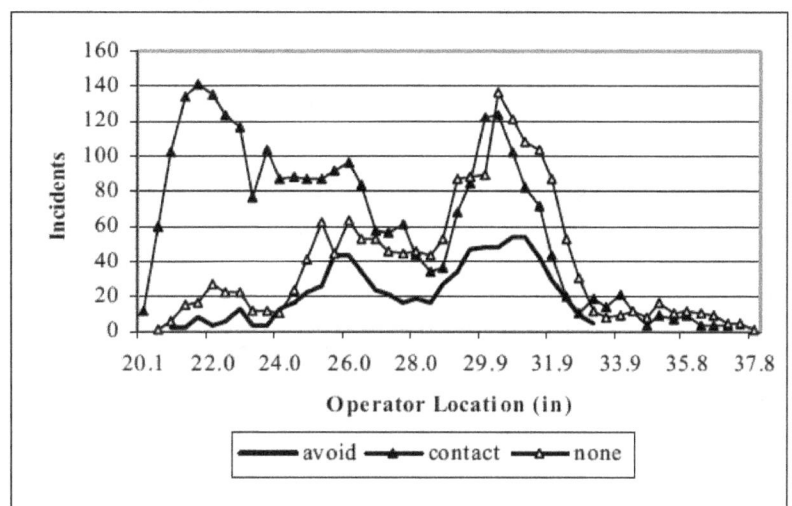

Table B 1.   Incidents by operator location

Operator location (in)	Avoid	Contact	None	Total incidents	Operator location (in)	Avoid	Contact	None	Total incidents
20.1	0	12	0	12	29.5	47	85	88	220
20.5	0	60	1	61	29.9	48	122	90	260
20.9	2	102	6	110	30.3	48	123	137	308
21.3	2	134	15	151	30.7	54	102	121	277
21.7	8	141	16	165	31.1	54	82	108	244
22.0	4	135	27	166	31.5	42	72	104	218
22.4	6	124	22	152	31.9	29	43	87	159
22.8	13	117	22	152	32.3	19	20	53	92
23.2	4	76	12	92	32.7	9	11	31	51
23.6	4	104	12	120	33.1	5	19	12	36
24.0	13	87	11	111	33.5	0	14	8	22
24.4	17	88	23	128	33.9	0	21	10	31
24.8	22	87	41	150	34.3	0	12	12	24
25.2	26	87	62	175	34.6	0	4	8	12
25.6	43	92	45	180	35.0	0	10	16	26
26.0	43	97	64	204	35.4	0	7	11	18
26.4	34	83	53	170	35.8	0	9	12	21
26.8	24	58	53	135	36.2	0	4	11	15
27.2	21	56	46	123	36.6	0	3	9	12
27.6	17	61	45	123	37.0	0	3	5	8
28.0	19	43	46	108	37.4	0	0	5	5
28.3	17	34	44	95	37.8	0	1	1	2
28.7	27	37	53	117	TOTAL	755	2,750	1,745	5,250
29.1	34	68	87	189					

32

Figure B 2.   Contact incidents by operator location and body part.

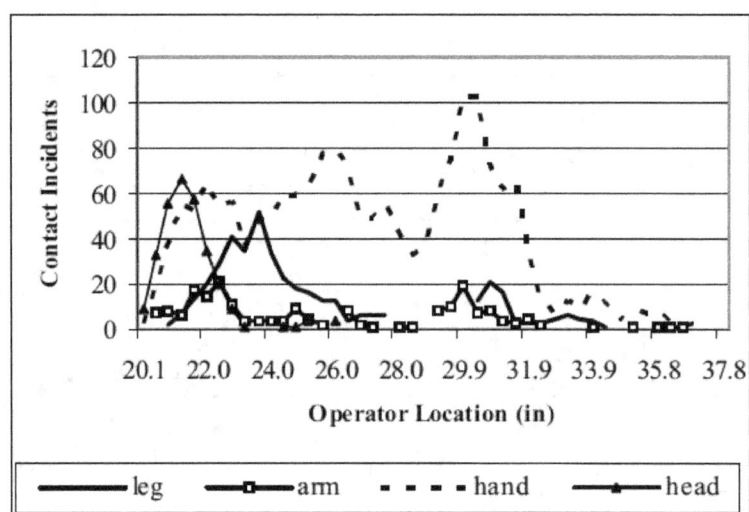

Table B 2.   Contact incidents by operator location and body part

Operator location (in)	Body part				Total contact incidents	Operator location (in)	Body part				Total contact incidents
	Leg	Arm	Hand	Head			Leg	Arm	Hand	Head	
20.1	0	0	3	9	12	29.5	0	10	75	0	85
20.5	0	7	20	33	60	29.9	0	19	103	0	122
20.9	2	8	37	55	102	30.3	13	7	103	0	123
21.3	7	6	55	66	134	30.7	21	8	73	0	102
21.7	14	17	53	57	141	31.1	16	4	62	0	82
22.0	20	15	65	35	135	31.5	3	3	66	0	72
22.4	29	21	54	20	124	31.9	3	5	35	0	43
22.8	41	11	56	9	117	32.3	3	2	15	0	20
23.2	35	4	36	1	76	32.7	5	0	6	0	11
23.6	52	4	48	0	104	33.1	6	0	13	0	19
24.0	34	4	49	0	87	33.5	5	0	9	0	14
24.4	23	4	60	1	88	33.9	4	1	16	0	21
24.8	18	9	59	1	87	34.3	1	0	11	0	12
25.2	16	5	62	4	87	34.6	0	0	4	0	4
25.6	13	2	77	0	92	35.0	0	1	9	0	10
26.0	13	0	80	4	97	35.4	0	0	7	0	7
26.4	4	8	71	0	83	35.8	0	1	8	0	9
26.8	6	2	50	0	58	36.2	0	1	3	0	4
27.2	6	1	49	0	56	36.6	0	1	2	0	3
27.6	6	0	55	0	61	37.0	0	0	3	0	3
28.0	0	1	42	0	43	37.4	0	0	0	0	0
28.3	0	1	33	0	34	37.8	0	0	1	0	1
28.7	0	0	37	0	37	TOTAL	419	201	1,835	295	2,750
29.1	0	8	60	0	68						

Figure B 3. Contact incidents by operator location and work posture.

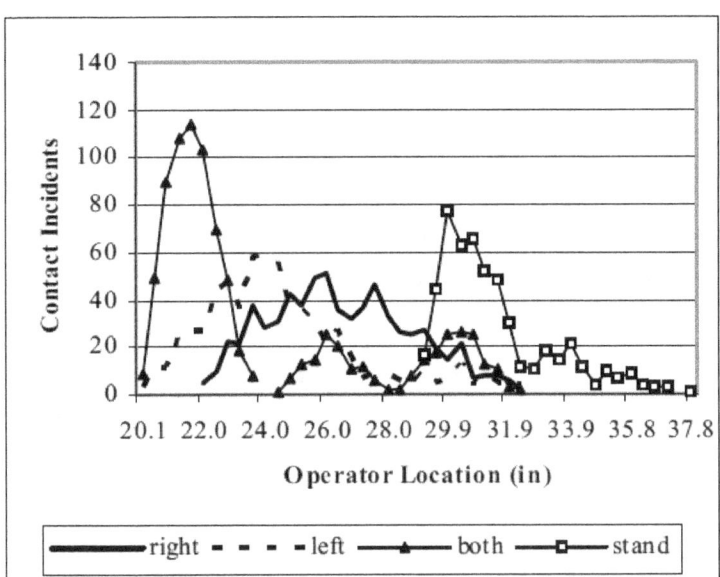

Table B 3. Contact incidents by operator location and work posture

Operator location (in)	Work posture				Total contact incidents	Operator location (in)	Work posture				Total contact incidents
	Right knee	Left knee	Both knees	Standing			Right knee	Left knee	Both knees	Standing	
20.1	0	3	9	0	12	29.5	19	5	17	44	85
20.5	0	11	49	0	60	29.9	14	6	25	77	122
20.9	0	12	90	0	102	30.3	21	13	26	63	123
21.3	0	26	108	0	134	30.7	7	4	25	66	102
21.7	0	27	114	0	141	31.1	8	9	13	52	82
22.0	5	27	103	0	135	31.5	8	5	11	48	72
22.4	10	44	70	0	124	31.9	6	4	3	30	43
22.8	22	47	48	0	117	32.3	2	4	2	12	20
23.2	21	37	18	0	76	32.7	0	0	0	11	11
23.6	38	58	8	0	104	33.1	0	1	0	18	19
24.0	28	59	0	0	87	33.5	0	0	0	14	14
24.4	31	56	1	0	88	33.9	0	0	0	21	21
24.8	42	38	7	0	87	34.3	0	0	0	12	12
25.2	38	36	13	0	87	34.6	0	0	0	4	4
25.6	49	29	14	0	92	35.0	0	0	0	10	10
26.0	51	21	25	0	97	35.4	0	0	0	7	7
26.4	36	27	20	0	83	35.8	0	0	0	9	9
26.8	32	15	11	0	58	36.2	0	0	0	4	4
27.2	37	7	12	0	56	36.6	0	0	0	3	3
27.6	46	9	6	0	61	37.0	0	0	0	3	3
28.0	33	8	2	0	43	37.4	0	0	0	0	0
28.3	26	6	2	0	34	37.8	0	0	0	1	1
28.7	25	4	8	0	37	TOTAL	682	669	874	525	2,750
29.1	27	11	14	16	68						

Figure B 4. Contact incidents by operator location and seam height.

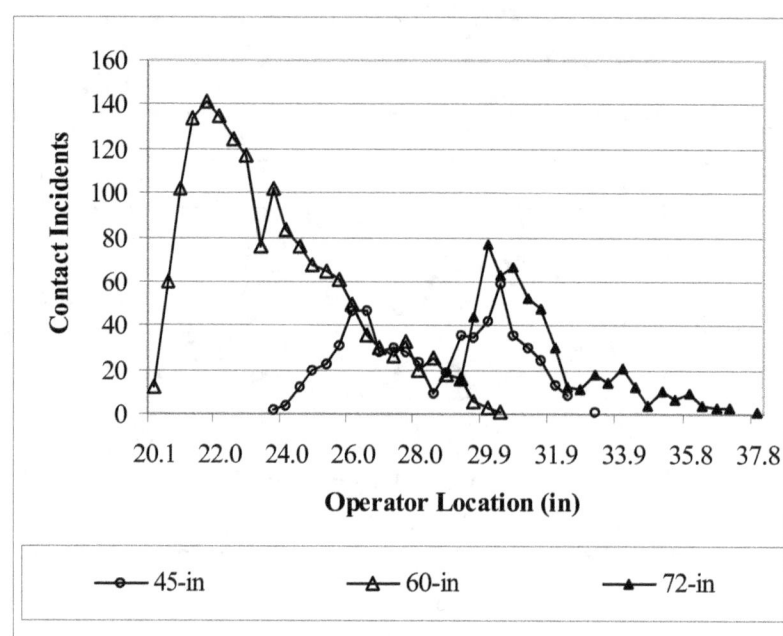

Table B 4. Contact incidents by operator location and seam height

Operator location (in)	Seam height (in)			Total contact incidents	Operator location (in)	Seam height (in)			Total contact incidents
	45	60	72			45	60	72	
20.1	0	12	0	12	29.5	35	6	44	85
20.5	0	60	0	60	29.9	42	3	77	122
20.9	0	102	0	102	30.3	59	1	63	123
21.3	0	134	0	134	30.7	36	0	66	102
21.7	0	141	0	141	31.1	30	0	52	82
22.0	0	135	0	135	31.5	24	0	48	72
22.4	0	124	0	124	31.9	13	0	30	43
22.8	0	117	0	117	32.3	8	0	12	20
23.2	0	76	0	76	32.7	0	0	11	11
23.6	2	102	0	104	33.1	1	0	18	19
24.0	4	83	0	87	33.5	0	0	14	14
24.4	12	76	0	88	33.9	0	0	21	21
24.8	20	67	0	87	34.3	0	0	12	12
25.2	22	65	0	87	34.6	0	0	4	4
25.6	31	61	0	92	35.0	0	0	10	10
26.0	47	50	0	97	35.4	0	0	7	7
26.4	47	36	0	83	35.8	0	0	9	9
26.8	28	30	0	58	36.2	0	0	4	4
27.2	30	26	0	56	36.6	0	0	3	3
27.6	28	33	0	61	37.0	0	0	3	3
28.0	23	20	0	43	37.4	0	0	0	0
28.3	9	25	0	34	37.8	0	0	1	1
28.7	19	18	0	37	TOTAL	606	1,619	525	2,750
29.1	36	16	16	68					

APPENDIX C.—FREQUENCY DATA SETS

Table C 1. Frequencies by data sets sorted by contacts

Conditions[1]	Frequencies				Percentages		
	Avoid incidents	Contacts	None	Total	Avoid incidents	Contacts	None
6022B	0	136	14	150	0.0	90.7	9.3
6016B	0	127	23	150	0.0	84.7	15.3
6010B	8	122	20	150	5.3	81.3	13.3
6007B	9	119	22	150	6.0	79.3	14.7
6007L	3	119	28	150	2.0	79.3	18.7
6022L	13	115	22	150	8.7	76.7	14.7
7213S	0	115	35	150	0.0	76.7	23.3
6013B	9	113	28	150	6.0	75.3	18.7
6022R	10	111	29	150	6.7	74.0	19.3
7210S	0	108	42	150	0.0	72.0	28.0
7216S	2	106	42	150	1.3	70.7	28.0
6016L	14	105	31	150	9.3	70.0	20.7
6016R	5	105	40	150	3.3	70.0	26.7
7207S	1	104	45	150	0.7	69.3	30.0
6010L	20	101	29	150	13.3	67.3	19.3
6013R	15	95	40	150	10.0	63.3	26.7
7222S	3	92	55	150	2.0	61.3	36.7
6013L	28	91	31	150	18.7	60.7	20.7
6010R	21	83	46	150	14.0	55.3	30.7
4516B	31	77	42	150	20.7	51.3	28.0
6007R	30	77	43	150	20.0	51.3	28.7
4516R	28	54	68	150	18.7	36.0	45.3
4507B	47	53	50	150	31.3	35.3	33.3
4513B	44	49	57	150	29.3	32.7	38.0
4522B	35	49	66	150	23.3	32.7	44.0
4522R	28	44	78	150	18.7	29.3	52.0
4507R	26	43	81	150	17.3	28.7	54.0
4513R	24	43	83	150	16.0	28.7	55.3
4516L	26	37	87	150	17.3	24.7	58.0
4513L	37	36	77	150	24.7	24.0	51.3
4522L	33	31	86	150	22.0	20.7	57.3
4510B	61	29	60	150	40.7	19.3	40.0
4510R	50	27	73	150	33.3	18.0	48.7
4507L	31	18	101	150	20.7	12.0	67.3
4510L	63	16	71	150	42.0	10.7	47.3
Total	755	2,750	1,745	5,250			

[1]The first two digits represent coal seam height (in). The second two digits represent boom arm speed (in/sec). The letter represents work posture as follows: R = right knee; L = left knee; B = both knees; S = standing.

Table C 2. Frequencies by data sets sorted by avoid incidents

Conditions[1]	Frequencies				Percentages		
	Avoid incidents	Contacts	None	Total	Avoid incidents	Contacts	None
4510L	63	16	71	150	42.0	10.7	47.3
4510B	61	29	60	150	40.7	19.3	40.0
4510R	50	27	73	150	33.3	18.0	48.7
4507B	47	53	50	150	31.3	35.3	33.3
4513B	44	49	57	150	29.3	32.7	38.0
4513L	37	36	77	150	24.7	24.0	51.3
4522B	35	49	66	150	23.3	32.7	44.0
4522L	33	31	86	150	22.0	20.7	57.3
4516B	31	77	42	150	20.7	51.3	28.0
4507L	31	18	101	150	20.7	12.0	67.3
6007R	30	77	43	150	20.0	51.3	28.7
6013L	28	91	31	150	18.7	60.7	20.7
4516R	28	54	68	150	18.7	36.0	45.3
4522R	28	44	78	150	18.7	29.3	52.0
4507R	26	43	81	150	17.3	28.7	54.0
4516L	26	37	87	150	17.3	24.7	58.0
4513R	24	43	83	150	16.0	28.7	55.3
6010R	21	83	46	150	14.0	55.3	30.7
6010L	20	101	29	150	13.3	67.3	19.3
6013R	15	95	40	150	10.0	63.3	26.7
6016L	14	105	31	150	9.3	70.0	20.7
6022L	13	115	22	150	8.7	76.7	14.7
6022R	10	111	29	150	6.7	74.0	19.3
6007B	9	119	22	150	6.0	79.3	14.7
6013B	9	113	28	150	6.0	75.3	18.7
6010B	8	122	20	150	5.3	81.3	13.3
6016R	5	105	40	150	3.3	70.0	26.7
6007L	3	119	28	150	2.0	79.3	18.7
7222S	3	92	55	150	2.0	61.3	36.7
7216S	2	106	42	150	1.3	70.7	28.0
7207S	1	104	45	150	0.7	69.3	30.0
6022B	0	136	14	150	0.0	90.7	9.3
6016B	0	127	23	150	0.0	84.7	15.3
7213S	0	115	35	150	0.0	76.7	23.3
7210S	0	108	42	150	0.0	72.0	28.0
Total	755	2,750	1,745	5,250			

[1]The first two digits represent coal seam height (in). The second two digits represent boom arm speed (in/sec). The letter represents work posture as follows: R = right knee; L = left knee; B = both knees; S = standing.

Table C 3. Data sets by body part and contacts

Conditions[1]	Body part				Total
	Leg	Arm	Hand	Head	
4507B		2	90	8	100
4507L		1	48		49
4507R		2	67		69
4510B		3	84	3	90
4510L			79		79
4510R		6	71		77
4513B		8	79	6	93
4513L		5	68		73
4513R		8	59		67
4516B		8	90	10	108
4516L		2	61		63
4516R		4	78		82
4522B		9	65	11	85
4522L		1	63		64
4522R		4	68		72
6007B		21	65	42	128
6007L	46	1	80		127
6007R	41	2	64		107
6010B		14	63	53	130
6010L	66	8	58		132
6010R	32	5	67		104
6013B		17	58	47	122
6013L	70	2	54		126
6013R	24		86		110
6016B		12	66	49	127
6016L	43	2	76		121
6016R	27	3	81		111
6022B		7	35	94	136
6022L	41	16	72		129
6022R	28	6	90		124
7207S	20	3	123		146
7210S	16	16	79		111
7213S	7	1	67		75
7216S	26	23	64		113
7222S	26	17	56		99
TOTAL	513	239	2,474	323	3,549

[1]The first two digits represent coal seam height (in). The second two digits represent boom arm speed (in/sec). The letter represents work posture as follows: R = right knee; L = left knee; B = both knees; S = standing.

APPENDIX D.—CROSS-TABULATION

Figure D 1. Contact incidents by seam height and boom direction.

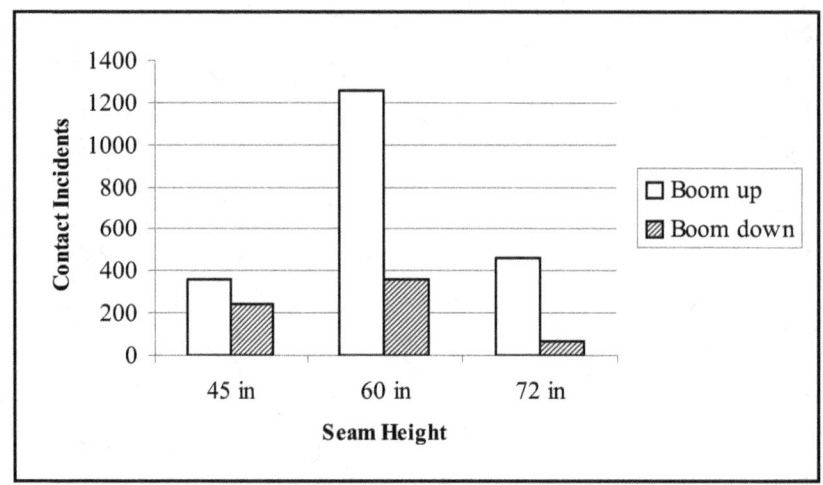

Table D 1. Contact incidents by seam height and boom direction

| Seam height, in | Boom direction | | Total | Summary[1] |
	Up	Down		
45	361	245	606	U>D
60	1,258	361	1,619	U>D
72	460	65	525	U>D
Total	2,079	671	2,750	

[1]D = down; U = up.

Figure D 2. Contact incidents by seam height and body part.

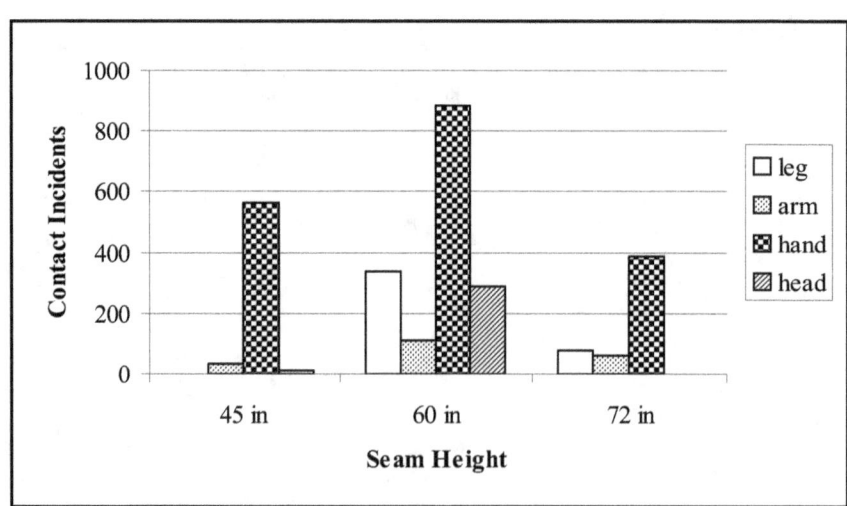

Table D 2. Contact incidents by seam height and body part

| Seam height, in | Body part | | | | Total | Summary[1] |
	Leg	Arm	Hand	Head		
45	0	33	563	10	606	H>A>HD>L
60	339	109	886	285	1,619	H>L>HD>A
72	80	59	386	0	525	H>L>A>HD
Total . . .	419	201	1,835	295	2,750	

[1]H = hand; A = arm; HD = head; L = leg.

Figure D 3. Contact incidents by seam height and machine part.

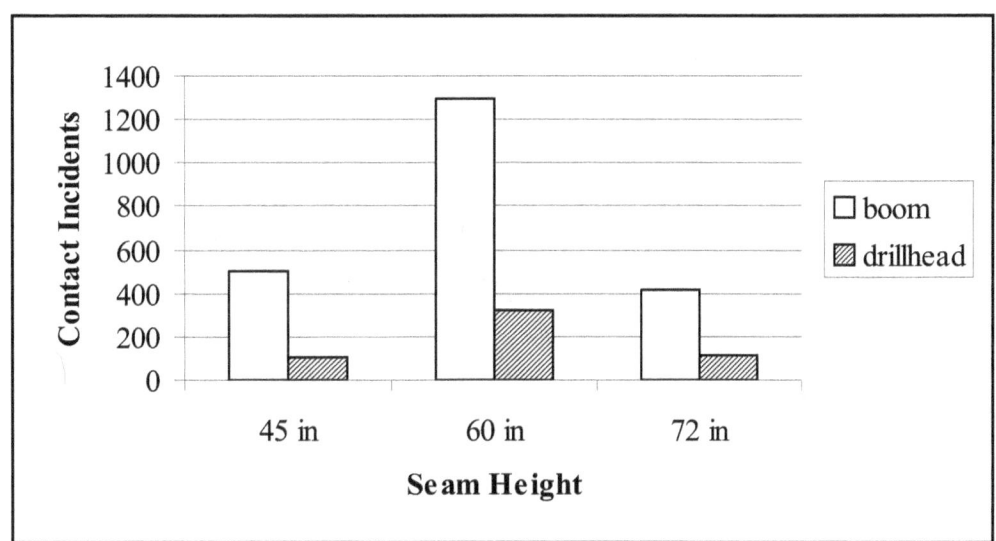

Table D 3. Contact incidents by seam height and machine part

Seam height, in	Machine part		Total	Summary[1]
	Boom	Drill head		
45	501	105	606	B>D
60	1,295	324	1,619	B>D
72	413	112	525	B>D
Total	2,209	541	2,750	

[1]B = boom; D = drill head.

Figure D 4. Contact incidents by operator percentile and boom direction.

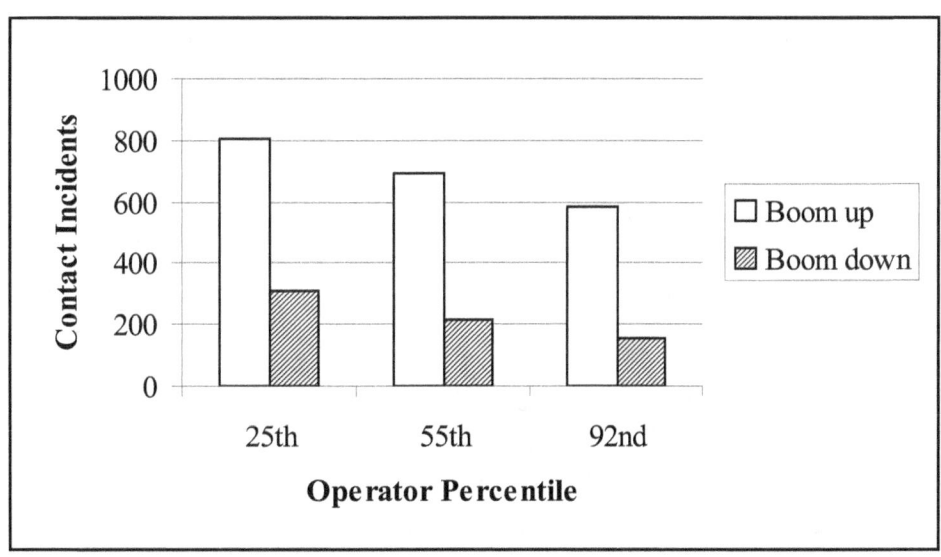

Table D 4. Contact incidents by operator percentile and boom direction

Operator percentile	Boom direction		Total	Summary[1]
	Up	Down		
25th	806	307	1,113	U>D
55th	688	212	900	U>D
92nd	585	152	737	U>D
Total	2,079	671	2,750	

[1]U = up; D = down.

Figure D 5. Contact incidents by operator percentile and body part.

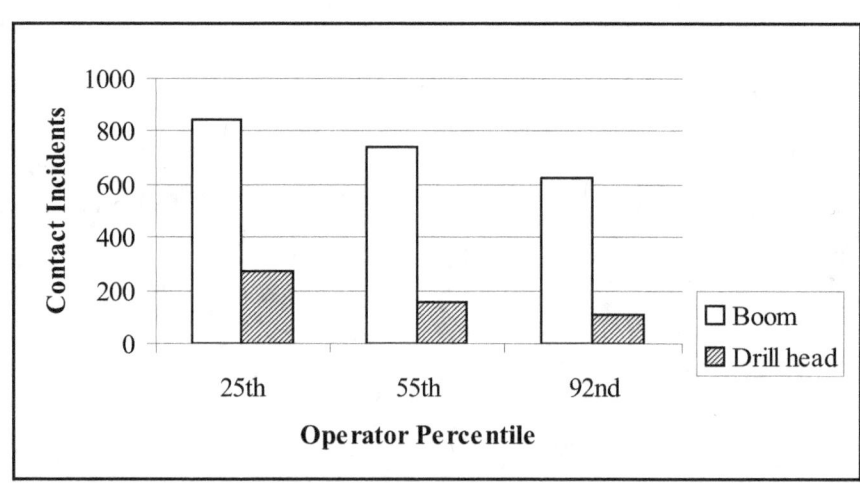

Table D 5. Contact incidents by operator percentile and body part

Operator percentile	Body part				Total	Summary[1]
	Leg	Arm	Hand	Head		
25th	158	117	753	85	1,113	H>L>A>HD
55th	181	60	578	81	900	H>L>HD>A
92nd	80	24	504	129	737	H>HD>L>A
Total	419	201	1,835	295	2,750	

[1]H = hand; L = leg; A = arm; HD = head.

Figure D 6. Contact incidents by operator percentile and machine part.

Table D 6. Contact incidents by operator percentile and machine part

Operator percentile	Machine part		Total	Summary[1]
	Boom	Drill head		
25th	841	272	1,113	B>D
55th	741	159	900	B>D
92nd	627	110	737	B>D
Total	2,209	541	2,750	

[1]B = boom; D = drill head.

Figure D 7. Contact incidents by work posture and boom direction.

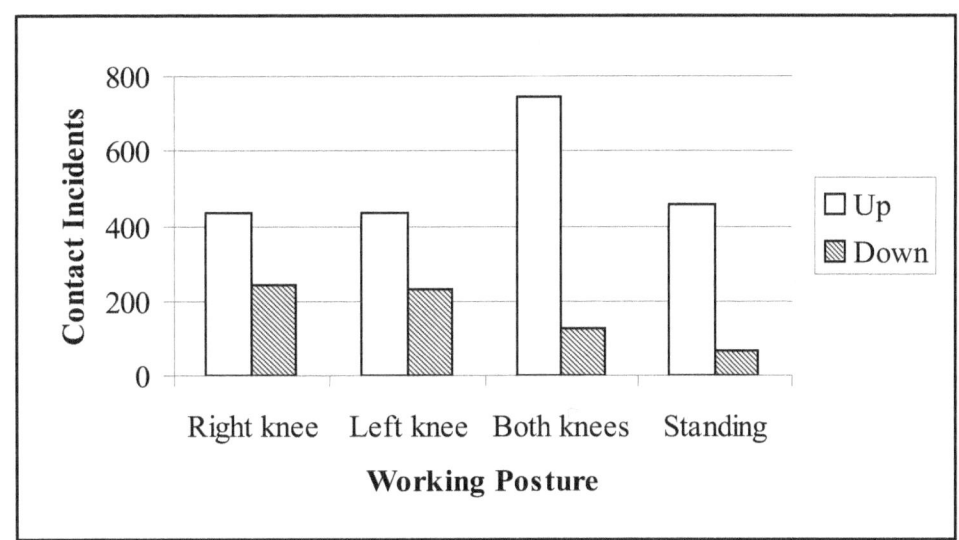

Table D 7. Contact incidents by work posture and boom direction

Work posture	Boom direction		Total	Summary[1]
	Down	Up		
Right knee	245	437	682	U>D
Left knee	233	436	669	U>D
Both knees	128	746	874	U>D
Standing	65	460	525	U>D
Total	671	2,079	2,750	

[1]U = up; D = down.

Figure D-8. Contact incidents by work posture and body part.

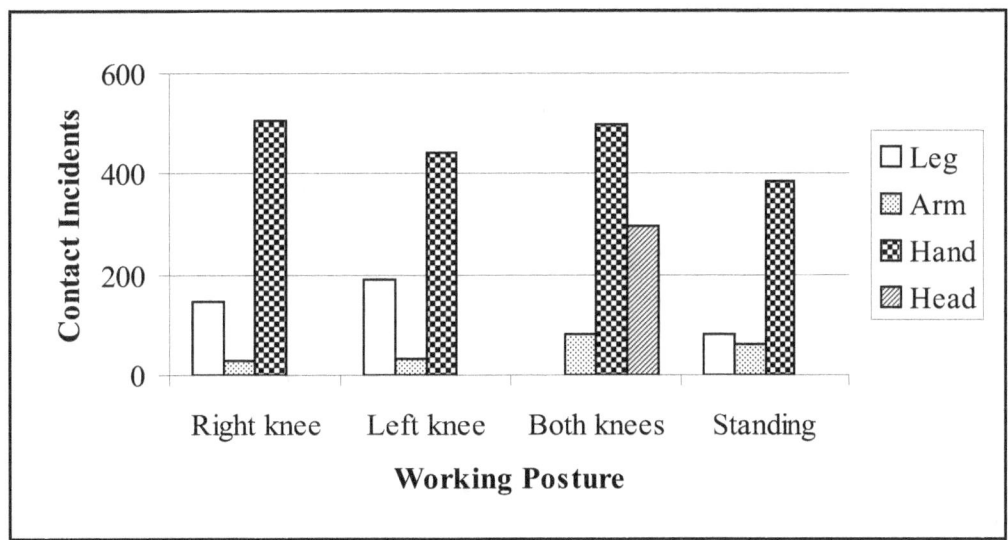

Table D 8. Contact incidents by work posture and body part

Work posture	Body part				Total	Summary[1]
	Leg	Arm	Hand	Head		
Right knee	147	28	507	0	682	H>L>A>HD
Left knee	192	34	443	0	669	H>L>A>HD
Both knees	0	80	499	295	874	H>HD>A>L
Standing	80	59	386	0	525	H>L>A>HD
Total	419	201	1,835	295	2,750	

[1]H = hand; L = leg; A = arm; HD = head.

Figure D 9.   Contact incidents by work posture and machine part.

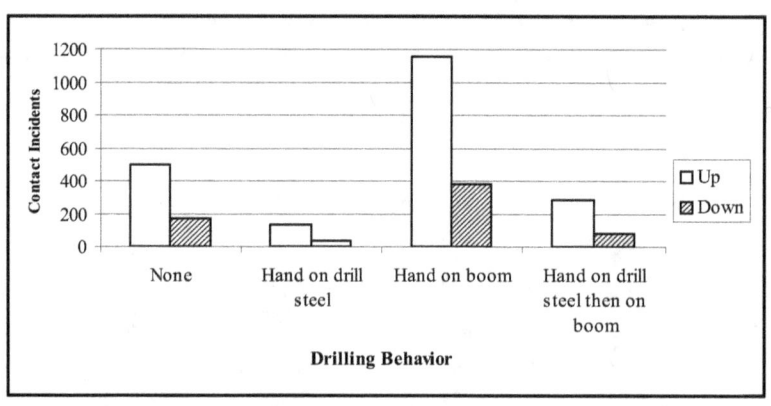

Table D 9.   Contact incidents by work posture and machine part

Work posture	Machine part		Total	Summary
	Boom	Drill head		
Right knee	563	119	682	B>D
Left knee	535	134	669	B>D
Both knees	698	176	874	B>D
Standing	413	112	525	B>D
Total	2,209	541	2,750	

[1]B = boom; D = drill head.

Figure D 10.   Contact incidents by drilling behavior and boom direction.

Table D 10.   Contact incidents by drilling behavior and boom direction

Drilling behavior	Boom direction		Total	Summary
	Up	Down		
None	501	172	673	U>D
Hand on drill steel	133	35	168	U>D
Hand on boom	1,160	381	1,541	U>D
Hand on drill steel then on boom .	285	83	368	U>D
Total	2,079	671	2,750	

[1]U = up; D = down.

Figure D 11. Contact incidents by drilling behavior and body part.

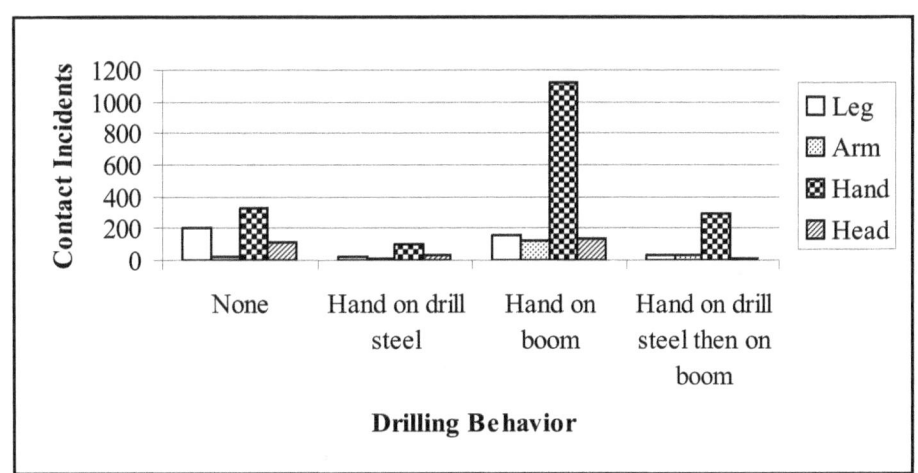

Table D 11. Contact incidents by drilling behavior and body part

Drilling behavior	Body part				Total	Summary[1]
	Leg	Arm	Hand	Head		
None	200	27	332	114	673	H>L>HD>A
Hand on drill steel	28	13	97	30	168	H>L>HD>A
Hand on boom	162	128	1,116	135	1,541	H>L>A>HD
Hand on drill steel then on boom .	29	33	290	16	368	H>A>L>HD
Total	419	201	1,835	295	2,750	

[1]H = hand; L = leg; HD = head; A = arm.

Figure D 12. Contact incidents by drilling behavior and machine part.

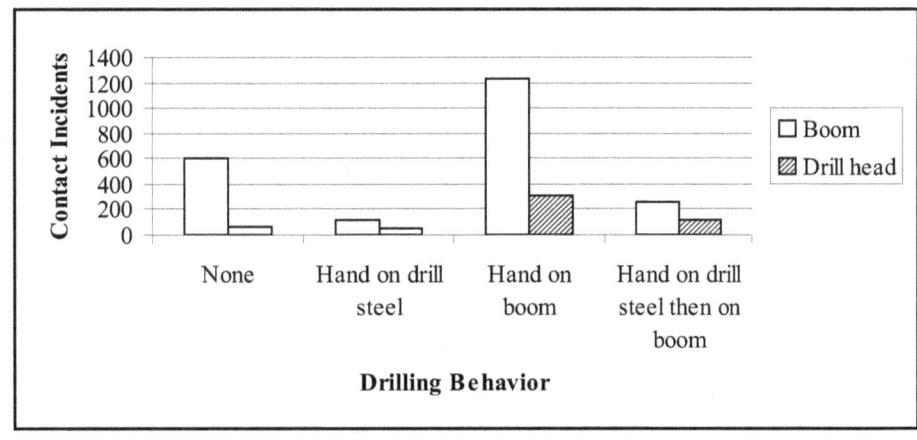

Table D 12. Contact incidents by drilling behavior and machine part

Drilling behavior	Machine part		Total	Summary[1]
	Boom	Drill head		
None	608	65	673	B>D
Hand on drill steel	111	57	168	B>D
Hand on boom	1,234	307	1,541	B>D
Hand on drill steel then on boom . . .	256	112	368	B>D
Total	2,209	541	2,750	

[1]B = boom; D = drill head.

Figure D 13. Contact incidents by bolting behavior and machine part.

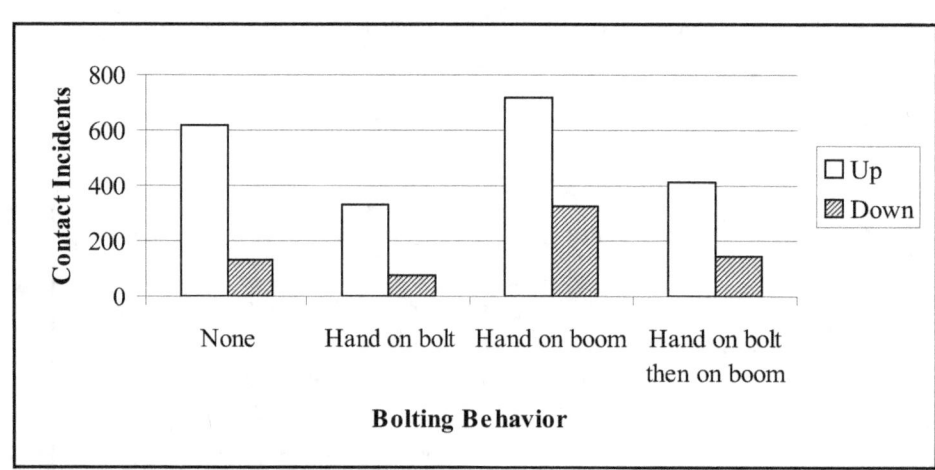

Table D 13. Contact incidents by bolting behavior and machine part

Bolting behavior	Machine part		Total	Summary[1]
	Boom	Drill head		
None	595	153	748	B>D
Hand on bolt	305	97	402	B>D
Hand on boom	870	172	1,042	B>D
Hand on bolt then on boom .	439	119	558	B>D
Total	2,209	541	2,750	

[1]B = boom; D = drill head.

Figure D 14. Contact incidents by bolting behavior and boom direction.

Table D 14. Contact incidents by bolting behavior and boom direction

Bolting behavior	Boom direction		Total	Summary
	Up	Down		
None	619	129	748	U>D
Hand on bolt	330	72	402	U>D
Hand on boom	716	326	1,042	U>D
Hand on bolt then on boom	414	144	558	U>D
Total	2,079	671	2,750	

[1]U = up; D = down.

Figure D 15. Contact incidents by bolting behavior and body part.

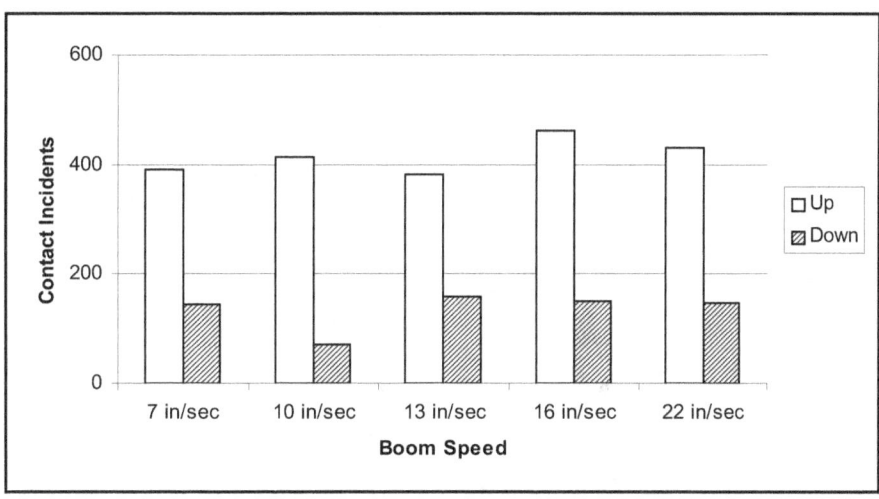

Table D 15. Contact incidents by bolting behavior and body part

Bolting behavior	Body part				Total	Summary[1]
	Leg	Arm	Hand	Head		
None	141	54	454	99	748	H>L>HD>A
Hand on bolt	67	41	237	57	402	H>L>HD>A
Hand on boom	143	69	738	92	1,042	H>L>HD>A
Hand on bolt then on boom .	68	37	406	47	558	H>L>HD>A
Total	419	201	1,835	295	2,750	

[1]H = hand; L = leg; HD = head; A = arm.

Figure D 16. Contact incidents by boom speed and boom direction.

Table D 16. Contact incidents by boom speed and boom direction

Boom speed, in/sec	Boom direction		Total	Summary
	Up	Down		
7	390	143	533	U>D
10	414	72	486	U>D
13	383	159	542	U>D
16	461	150	611	U>D
22	431	147	578	U>D
Total	2,079	671	2,750	

[1]U = up; D = down.

Figure D 17. Contact incidents by boom speed and body part.

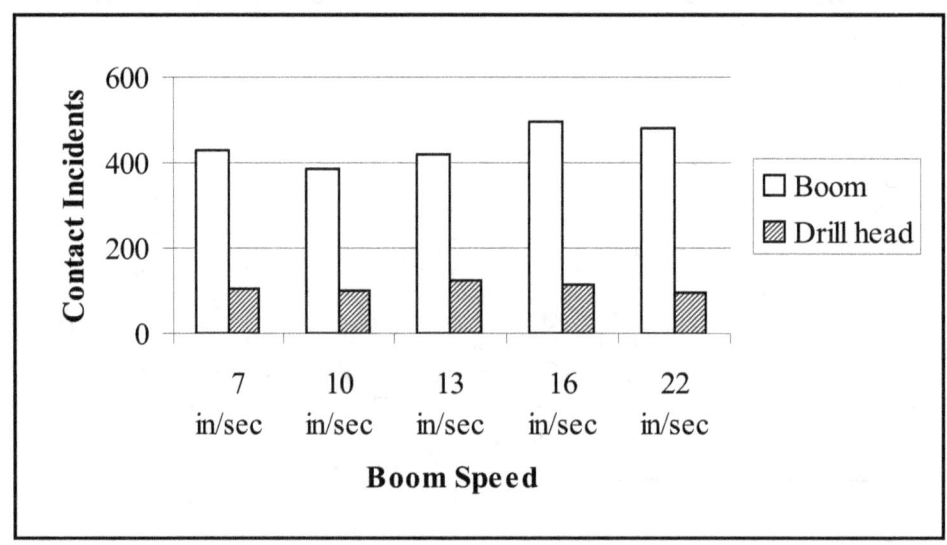

Table D 17. Contact incidents by boom speed and body part

Boom speed, in/sec	Body part				Total	Summary[1]
	Leg	Arm	Hand	Head		
7	99	25	359	50	533	H>L>HD>A
10	90	42	300	54	486	H>L>HD>A
13	76	31	387	48	542	H>L>HD>A
16	78	47	437	49	611	H>L>HD>A
22	76	56	352	94	578	H>HD>L>A
Total	419	201	1,835	295	2,750	

[1]H = hand; L = leg; HD = head; A = arm.

Figure D 18. Contact incidents by boom speed and machine part.

Table D 18. Contact incidents by boom speed and machine part

Boom speed, in/sec	Machine part		Total	Summary[1]
	Boom	Drill head		
7	428	105	533	B>D
10	384	102	486	B>D
13	420	122	542	B>D
16	496	115	611	B>D
22	481	97	578	B>D
Total	2,209	541	2,750	

[1]B = boom; D = drill head.

Figure D 19.   Contact incidents by boom speed and work posture.

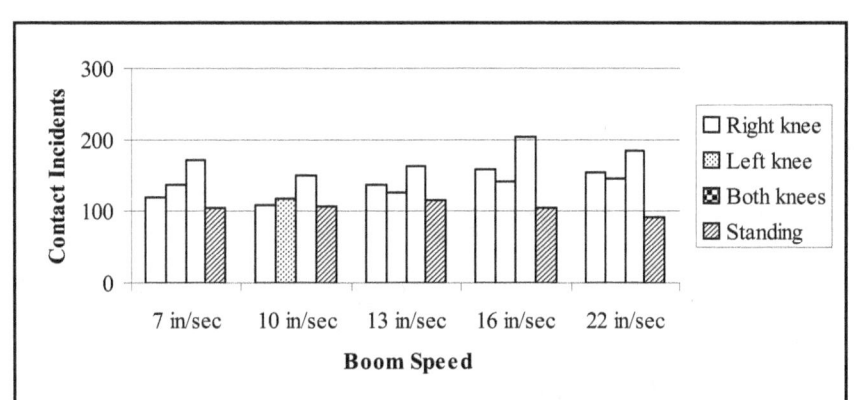

Table D 19.   Contact incidents by boom speed and work posture

Boom speed, in/sec	Work posture				Total	Summary[1]
	Right knee	Left knee	Both knees	Standing		
7	120	137	172	104	533	B>L>R>S
10	110	117	151	108	486	B>L>R>S
13	138	127	162	115	542	B>R>L>S
16	159	142	204	106	611	B>R>L>S
22	155	146	185	92	578	B>R>L>S
Total	682	669	874	525	2,750	

[1]L = left knee; R = right knee; B = both knees; S = standing.

Figure D 20.   Contact incidents by boom speed and operator percentile.

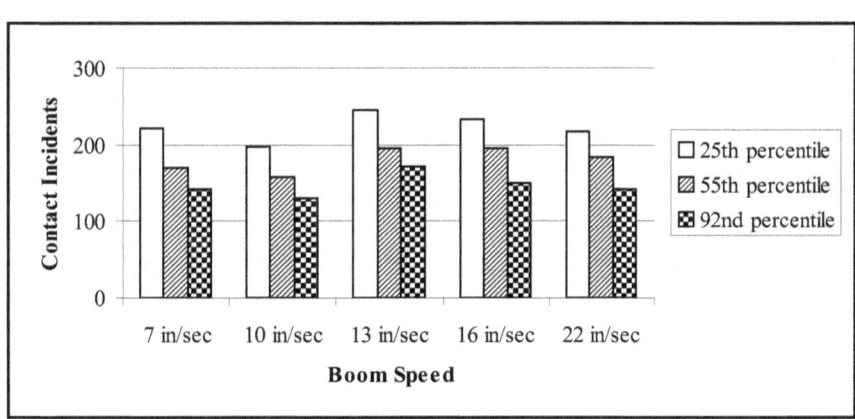

Table D 20.   Contact incidents by boom speed and operator percentile

Boom speed, in/sec	Operator percentile			Total	Summary
	25th	55th	92nd		
7	221	169	143	533	25>55>92
10	197	158	131	486	25>55>92
13	245	195	171	611	25>55>92
16	233	195	150	578	25>55>92
22	217	183	142	542	25>55>92
Total	1,113	900	737	2,750	

Figure D 21.   Contact incidents by boom speed and drilling behavior.

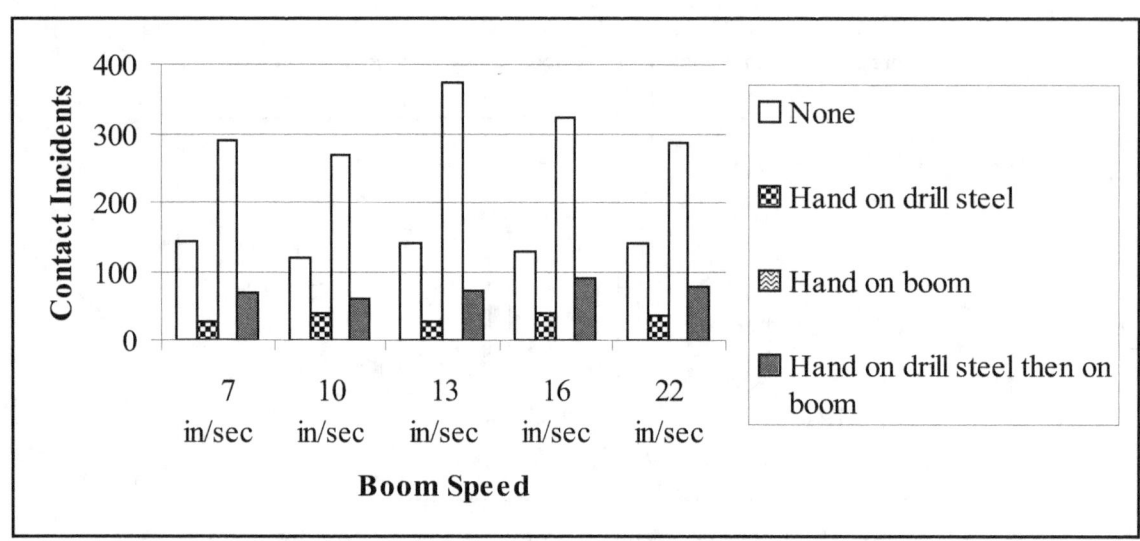

Table D 21.   Contact incidents by boom speed and drilling behavior

Boom speed, in/sec	Drilling behavior				Total	Summary[1]
	None	Hand on drill steel	Hand on boom	Hand on drill steel then on boom		
7	144	28	291	70	533	B>N>D&B>D
10	120	39	268	59	486	B>N>D&B>D
13	140	26	373	72	611	B>N>D&B>D
16	129	38	322	89	578	B>N>D&B>D
22	140	37	287	78	542	B>N>D&B>D
Total	673	168	1,541	368	2,750	

[1]D = hand on drill steel; B = hand on boom; D&B = hand on drill steel then on boom; N = none.

Figure D 22.   Contact incidents by boom speed and seam height.

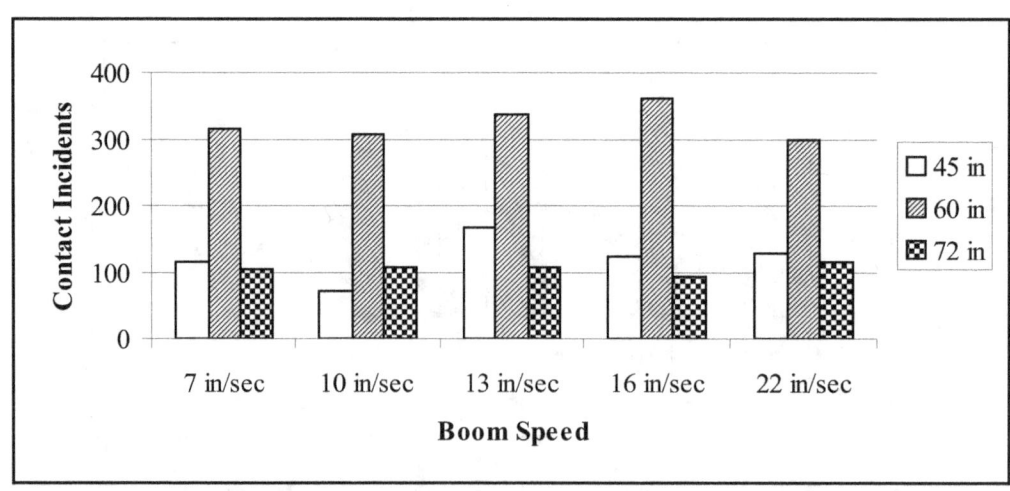

Table D 22.   Contact incidents by boom speed and seam height

Boom speed, in/sec	Seam height, in			Total	Summary
	45	60	72		
7	114	315	104	533	60>45>72
10	72	306	108	486	60>72>45
13	168	337	106	611	60>45>72
16	124	362	92	578	60>45>72
22	128	299	115	542	60>45>72
Total	606	1,619	525	2,750	

Figure D 23. Contact incidents by boom speed and bolting behavior.

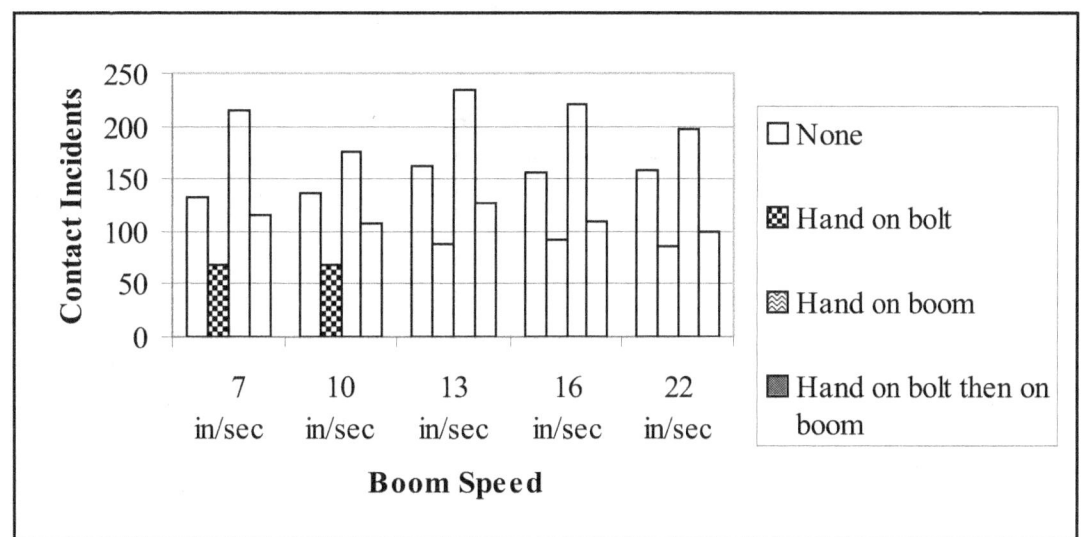

Table D 23. Contact incidents by boom speed and bolting behavior

Boom speed, in/sec	Bolting behavior				Total	Summary[1]
	None	Hand on bolt	Hand on boom	Hand on bolt then on boom		
7	133	69	215	116	533	B>N>BT&B>BT
10	136	68	175	107	486	B>N>BT&B>BT
13	163	88	234	126	611	B>N>BT&B>BT
16	157	91	220	110	578	B>N>BT&B>BT
22	159	86	198	99	542	B>N>BT&B>BT
Total	748	402	1,042	558	2,750	

[1]BT = hand on bolt; B = hand on boom; BT&B = hand on bolt then on boom; N = none.

APPENDIX E.—LOGISTIC REGRESSION MODELS FOR ROOF BOLTER SIMULATION DATA

Table E 1. Modeling the probability of a contact for slow reaction time of operator (N = 5,250)

Model	Predictor variable	β	SE(β)	Ψ	Pr > chi square	R^2
1	Seam height:					
	45 in			1.000		0.2435
	60 in	1.9403	0.0668	6.961	<.0001	
	72 in	1.8453	0.0928	6.330	<.0001	
2	Boom speed:					
	7 in/sec			1.000		0.0087
	10 in/sec	0.1793	0.0874	0.836	0.0402	
	13 in/sec	0.0343	0.0873	1.035	0.6944	
	16 in/sec	0.3301	0.0879	1.350	0.0006	
	22 in/sec	0.1721	0.0875	1.188	0.0492	
3	Operator percentile:					
	55th			1.000		0.0410
	25th	0.5020	0.0690	1.652	<.0001	
	92nd	0.3731	0.0681	0.689	<.0001	
4	Working posture:					
	Standing			1.000		0.0456
	Right knee	1.0287	0.0951	0.357	<.0001	
	Left knee	1.0637	0.0951	0.345	<.0001	
	Both knees	0.5132	0.0953	0.599	<.0001	
5	Working posture/seam height:					
	Standing/72 in			1.000		
	Right knee/45 in	1.8941	0.1176	0.150	<.0001	
	Right knee/60 in	0.3419	0.1129	0.710	0.0024	
	Left knee/45 in	2.4724	0.1274	0.084	<.0001	
	Left knee/60 in	0.0404	0.1161	1.041	0.7277	
	Both knees/45 in	1.5904	0.1144	0.204	<.0001	
	Both knees/60 in	0.7179	0.1272	2.050	<.0001	
	Boom speed:					
	7 in/sec			1.000		0.3195
	10 in/sec	0.2377	0.1007	0.788	0.0182	
	13 in/sec	0.0453	0.1007	1.046	0.6525	
	16 in/sec	0.3995	0.1015	1.491	<.0001	
	22 in/sec	0.2291	0.1010	1.257	<.0233	
	Operator percentile:					
	55th			1.000		
	25th	0.6553	0.0793	1.926	<.0001	
	92nd	0.4859	0.0777	0.615	<.0001	

APPENDIX F.—SURVIVAL ANALYSIS TABLES

Table F 1. Univariate model information (outcome slow)

Variable	Degrees of freedom	Beta	Standard error	p value	Risk ratio	95% confidence interval		AIC	Proportional hazards probability
Operator location	1	.012	.002	.000	0.988	0.984	0.992	39058.426	.274
Operator percentile:	2							39079.482	.857
55th........................		.016	.045	.723	1.016	0.930	1.110		
92nd		.167	.048	.001	1.181	1.075	1.298		
Boom speed:[1]	4							38431.442	.000
10 in/sec		.412	.065	.000	1.510	1.330	1.714		
13 in/sec		.741	.065	.000	2.098	1.847	2.383		
16 in/sec		1.266	.065	.000	3.547	3.12	4.032		
22 in/sec		1.507	.067	.000	4.514	3.956	5.150		
Boom up	1	0.832	.045	.000	2.297	2.104	2.508	38703.881	.000
Bolting behavior:	3							39035.802	.059
Hand on bolt		.187	.062	.003	.829	0.734	0.937		
Hand on boom		.344	.049	.000	.709	0.644	0.781		
Hand on bolt then on boom ...		.386	.057	.000	.692	0.619	0.774		
Drilling behavior:	3							38793.809	.000
Hand on drill steel		.524	.087	.000	1.688	1.424	2.001		
Hand on boom		.716	.048	.000	2.046	1.862	2.248		
Hand on drill steel then on boom		.961	.067	.000	2.613	2.292	2.980		
Work posture/seam height:	6							38892.369	.000
Right knee/45 in		.290	.083	.000	.748	.636	.881		
Right knee/60 in		.308	.065	.000	.735	.647	.835		
Left knee/45 in		.577	.097	.000	.562	.464	.680		
Left knee/60 in		.278	.063	.000	.757	.669	.857		
Both knees/45 in		.371	.078	.000	.690	.592	.804		
Both knees/60 in		.356	.061	.000	1.427	1.267	1.608		

[1]Variable whose selection at this step best improves model fit as determined by Akaike Information Criterion.

Table F 2. Models with boom speed

Variable	Degrees of freedom	Beta	Standard error	p value	Risk ratio	95% confidence interval		AIC	Proportional hazards probability
Operator position	1	.014	.002	.000	0.986	0.982	0.990	38318.271	0.000
Operator percentile:	2							38340.011	0.714
55th........................		.002	.045	.963	1.002	0.917	1.095		
92nd		.205	.048	.000	1.228	1.118	1.349		
Boom up[1]	1	0.860	.045	.000	2.363	2.719	3.486	37948.863	.000
Bolting behavior:	3							38284.763	.000
Hand on bolt		.236	.063	.000	.790	.698	.893		
Hand on boom		.401	.049	.000	.670	.608	.738		
Hand on bolt then on boom		.432	.057	.000	.649	.580	.726		
Drilling behavior:	3							37964.690	.000
Hand on drill steel		.583	.088	.000	1.791	1.508	2.128		
Hand on boom		.846	.049	.000	2.329	2.118	2.563		
Hand on drill steel then on boom ..		1.078	.067	.000	2.939	2.576	3.353		
Work posture/seam height:	6							38178.128	.000
Right knee/45 in		.078	.086	.365	.925	.781	1.095		
Right knee/60 in		.255	.067	.000	.775	.680	.884		
Left knee/45 in		.405	.100	.000	.667	.548	.810		
Left knee/60 in		.137	.065	.036	.872	.767	.991		
Both knees/45 in		.143	.081	.078	.867	.739	1.016		
Both knees/60 in		.484	.063	.000	1.623	1.435	1.836		

[1]Variable whose selection at this step best improves model fit as determined by Akaike Information Criterion.

Table F 3. Models with boom speed, boom direction

Variable	Degrees of freedom	Beta	Standard error	p value	Risk ratio	95% confidence interval		AIC	Proportional hazards probability
Operator location	1	.007	.002	.001	.734	.989	.997	37688.279	0.000
Operator percentile:	2							37682.262	0.461
25th........................		.008	.045	.865	1.008	.922	1.101		
92nd		.241	.048	.000	1.272	1.158	1.398		
Bolting behavior:	3							37641.491	0.000
Hand on bolt		.256	.063	.000	.774	.685	.875		
Hand on boom		.348	.050	.000	.706	.640	.779		
Hand on bolt then on boom		.452	.057	.000	.636	.569	.712		
Drilling behavior:[1]	3							37123.513	.000
Hand on drill steel		.636	.088	.000	1.889	1.591	2.243		
Hand on boom		1.025	.048	.000	2.788	2.536	3.064		
Hand on drill steel then on boom ..		1.266	.067	.000	3.546	3.109	4.045		
Work posture/seam height:	6							37581.826	0.000
Right knee/45 in		.476	.089	.000	1.609	1.352	1.916		
Right knee/60 in		.095	.067	.159	.909	.797	1.038		
Left knee/45 in		.202	.102	.049	1.223	1.001	1.495		
Left knee/60 in		.018	.066	.782	.982	.864	1.117		
Both knees/45 in		.047	.082	.561	1.049	.893	1.231		
Both knees/60 in		.492	.063	.000	1.636	1.446	1.851		

[1]Variable whose selection at this step best improves model fit as determined by Akaike Information Criterion.

Table F 4. Models with boom speed, boom direction, drilling behavior

Variable	Degrees of freedom	Beta	Standard error	p value	Risk ratio	95% confidence interval		AIC	Proportional hazards probability
Operator location	1	.013	.002	.000	.987			36928.749	.000
Operator percentile:	2							36948.790	.806
25th........................		.063	.045	.165	0.939	.859	1.026		
92nd		.166	.048	.001	1.181	1.074	1.299		
Bolting behavior:	3							36910.591	0.000
Hand on bolt		.184	.063	.004	.832	.735	.941		
Hand on boom		.323	.050	.000	.724	.656	.799		
Hand on bolt then on boom		.415	.057	.000	.661	.590	.739		
Work posture/seam height:[1]	6							36797.873	.000
Right knee/45 in		.444	.088	.000	1.558	1.310	1.853		
Right knee/60 in		.066	.068	.332	1.936	0.820	1.069		
Left knee/45 in		.250	.102	.014	1.284	1.051	1569		
Left knee/60 in		.059	.066	.372	1.060	0.932	1.206		
Both knees/45 in		.181	.082	.026	1.199	1.021	1.407		
Both knees/60 in		.658	.063	.000	1.930	1.705	2.185		

[1]Variable whose selection at this step best improves model fit as determined by Akaike Information Criterion.

Table F 5. Models with boom speed, boom direction, drilling behavior, work posture/seam height

Variable	Degrees of freedom	Beta	Standard error	p value	Risk ratio	95% confidence interval		AIC	Proportional hazards probability
Operator location	1	.006	.005	.170	.994	.985	1.003	36180.209	.492
Operator percentile:	2							36175.668	.979
25th........................		.054	.046	.241	0.948	.867	1.037		
92nd		.093	.049	.057	1.098	.997	1.208		
Bolting behavior:[1]	3							36122.493	.046
Hand on bolt		.162	.063	.010	.850	.751	.962		
Hand on boom		.321	.051	.000	.725	.657	.801		
Hand on bolt then on boom		.428	.058	.000	.652	.582	.731		

[1]Variable whose selection at this step best improves model fit as determined by Akaike Information Criterion.

Table F 6.   Models with boom speed, boom direction, drilling behavior, work posture/seam height, bolting behavior

Variable	Degrees of freedom	Beta	Standard error	p value	Risk ratio	95% confidence interval	AIC	Proportional hazards probability
Operator location	1	.002	.005	.588	.998	.989 1.007	36122.228	0.762
Operator percentile:[1]	2						36115.613	0.946
25th		.036	.046	.429	.964	.882 1.055		
92nd		.112	.049	.023	1.118	1.016 1.231		

[1]Variable whose selection at this step best improves model fit as determined by Akaike Information Criterion.

Table F 7.   Models with boom speed, boom direction, drilling behavior, work posture/seam height,
bolting behavior, operator percentile

Variable	Degrees of freedom	Beta	Standard error	p value	Risk ratio	95% confidence interval	AIC	Proportional hazards probability
Operator location[1]	1	.017	.007	.011	.983	.970 .996	36114.925	0.335

[1]Variable whose selection at this step best improves model fit as determined by Akaike Information Criterion.

Table F 8.   Final model

$h(t|z) = h_0(t|z)\exp($ $2.3*10in/s +1.173*10in/s*\ln(time)$

$3.698*13in/s + 1.971*13in/s*\ln(time)$

$3.89*16in/s + 2.299*16in/s*\ln(time)$

$4.234*22in/s + 2.649*22in/s*\ln(time) +$

$2.995*boomup$ $0.668*boomup*\ln(time) +$

$3.906*handondrillsteel(drill)$ $1.142*handondrillsteel(drill)*\ln(time) +$

$4.978*handonboom(drill)$ $1.428*handonboom(drill)*\ln(time)$

$5.282*handonboth(drill)$ $1.465*handonboth(drill)*\ln(time)$

$9.236*Right45in + 3.927*Right45in*\ln(time)$

$6.049*Right60in + 2.291*Right60in*\ln(time)$

$9.47*Left45in + 3.959*Left45in*\ln(time)$

$6.002*Left60in + 2.274*Left60in*\ln(time)$

$9.014*Both45in + 3.743*Both45in*\ln(time)$

$2.539*Both60in + 1.137*Both60in*\ln(time) +$

$0.675*handonbolt(bolt)$ $0.341*handonbolt(bolt) +$

$0.25*handonboom(bolt)$ $0.23*handonboom(bolt)*\ln(time) +$

$0.241*handonboth(bolt)$ $0.268*handonboth(bolt)*\ln(time) +$

$0.047*55^{th}percentile + 0.243*95^{th}percentile$ $0.170*operatorlocation)$

APPENDIX G.—ILLUSTRATIONS OF OPERATOR'S WORK BEHAVIORS

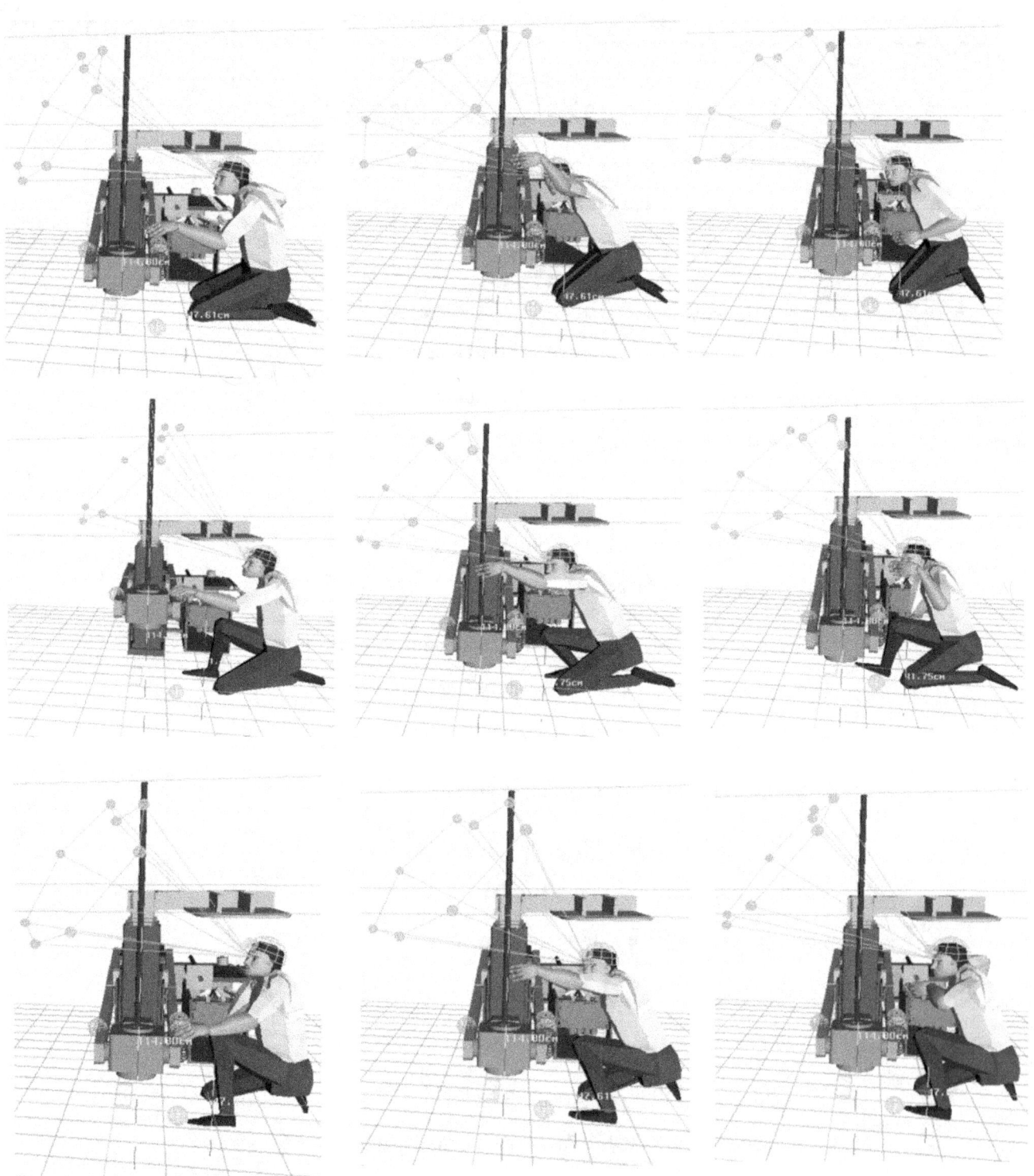

Figure G 1. 45-in seam height and different work postures: operator's hand on the boom arm, hand on the drill steel, hand off both boom arm and drill steel.

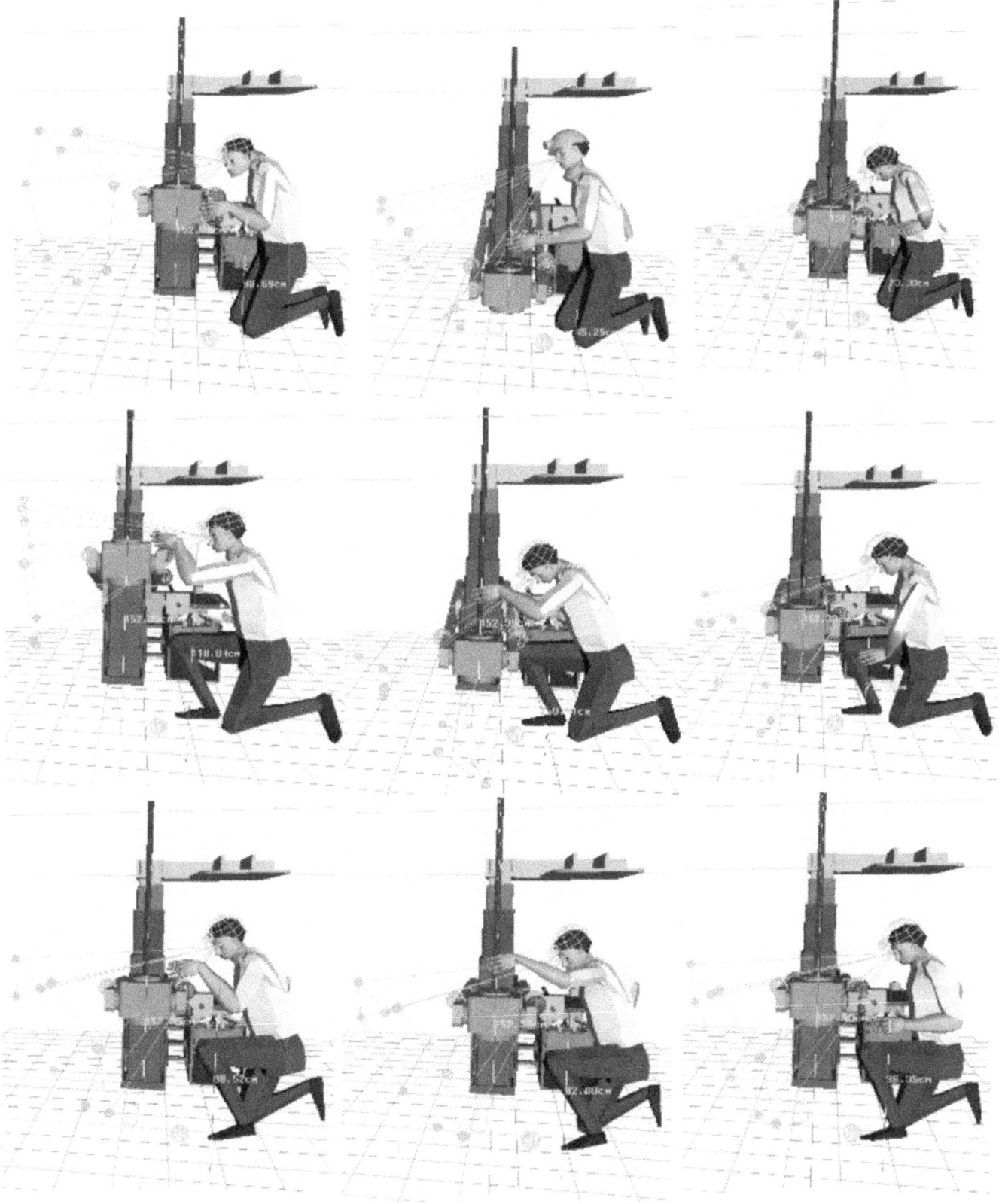

Figure G 2. 60-in seam height and different work postures: operator's hand on the boom arm, hand on the drill steel, hand off both boom arm and drill steel.

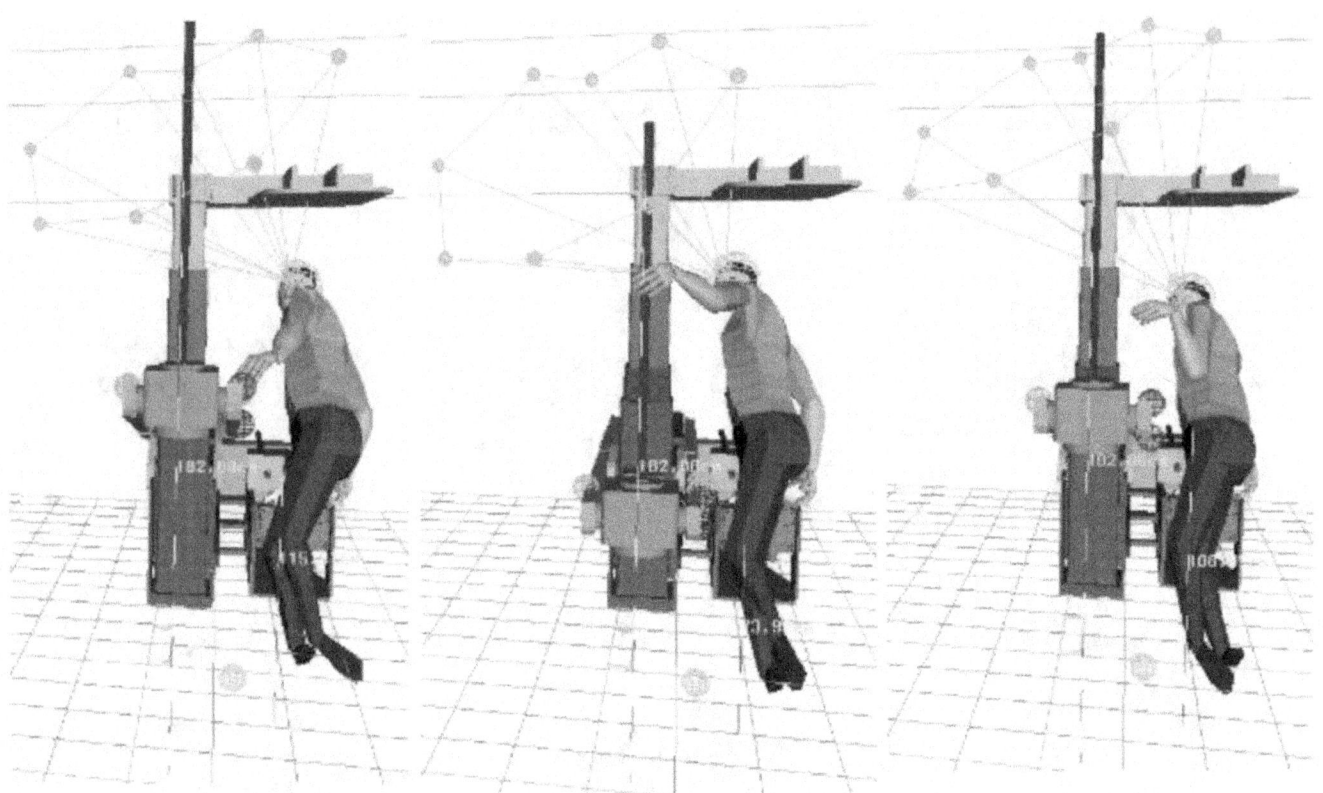

Figure G 3.   72-in seam height and standing work posture: operator's hand on the boom arm, hand on the drill steel, hand off both boom arm and drill steel.